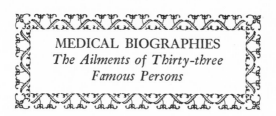

MEDICAL BIOGRAPHIES
*The Ailments of Thirty-three
Famous Persons*

MEDICAL BIOGRAPHIES

The Ailments of Thirty-three Famous Persons

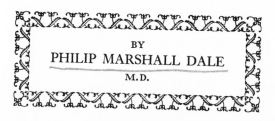

BY
PHILIP MARSHALL DALE
M.D.

FOREWORD BY
HOWARD F. STEIN

UNIVERSITY OF OKLAHOMA PRESS
NORMAN AND LONDON

LIBRARY OF CONGRESS CATALOGING-IN-PUBLICATION DATA

DALE, PHILIP MARSHALL, 1883–
MEDICAL BIOGRAPHIES.

BIBLIOGRAPHY: P.
INCLUDES INDEX.
1. CELEBRITIES—DISEASES. 2. CELEBRITIES—BIOGRAPHY.
3. MEDICINE—CASE STUDIES. 4. DISEASES AND HISTORY.
I. TITLE. [DNLM: 1. FAMOUS PERSONS—BIOGRAPHY.
WZ 313 D139M]
R703.D3   1987   920'.02   86-27209
ISBN 0–8061–2046–0 (PBK.)

To Bergette

FOREWORD

By Howard F. Stein

It can accurately be said that modern biomedicine takes disease out of life and sets it within its own technologically-dominated province. But then, to segregate disease from life is medicine's modern social role. In *Medical Biographies*, a work as refreshingly integrative today as when it was first published in 1952, P. M. Dale restores disease to the lives of those grand historical figures who suffered. Dale's achievement is greater than the modest claim he makes in his Preface: "To illumine a dark corner of legitimate biography, in a few select instances, with the light of modern medical understanding." He did, in fact, do that in the light of the medical knowledge of the early 1950s (thus making the book a historical document itself, as well as an account of historic figures). He has in his vignettes given a sketch of what it was like to be alive and ill and in treatment in a wide array of historical eras and cultures, described what some of the folk and official medical beliefs and practices were at various times, sketched the social views of sicknesses during different ages, and offered portraits of medicine itself in these various periods. Thus, while Dale succeeded in offering succinct biographical portraits of disease in the lives of famous persons of the past, he offered equally vivid pictures of the context as well.

As a medical anthropologist who has taught physicians and medical students for fifteen years in medical settings, I found Dale's narrative refreshing, a welcome departure from the often arid, antiseptic, even lifeless medical biographies which are recounted in case conferences and in medical charting. Far from anesthetizing the reader to decay, debilitation, decline, and death, Dale has made these his subject. While not espousing a psychosomatic or family-somatic or what is now called a biopsy-chosocial "systems" model of disease, Dale nonetheless shows how many of his protagonists' lives prepared them for the disease that afflicted them. It is a psychological irony— one which I more read into the text than infer was Dale's intention— that he describes the havoc diseases have wrought on men and women whom we (and they) had thought to control history and destiny!

As a teacher in medical school, I found the vignettes especially useful in understanding human suffering—an antidote to reducing suffering to disease entities. Dale's case vignettes attest to what it was like to live, fall ill, and die in a world—so different from our own of the 1980s—in which widespread fatal infectious disease was the rule rather than the exception. Yet the distinction between the times Dale writes about and our own should not be overdrawn: for just as the scourge of smallpox was eliminated in the 1980s, syphilis was once again on the rise, and the still mysterious AIDS malady was discovered. So much has AIDS captured the popular American imagination, as well as terrified current practitioners and researchers rushing to control if not conquer it, that were Dale composing his book anew today, AIDS would certainly have been included.

We have learned much since 1952 about the relationship between life and disease—a relationship already alluded to above. In their book, *The Psychological Autopsy*, Weisman and Kastenbaum (1968) draw the valuable distinction between the disease a person dies with and what that person dies from. When one strives to understand someone's medical biography, it is useful not to assume that disease or disability are automatically a departure from, or rude invasion into, that person's life themes and life course. The disease a person dies with may well be comprehended as an extension or culmination of those deeper personal and family struggles that have prepared the medium for the entry of the disease onto the historical stage. Diseases are real; they have effects on people's, families', and communities' lives. But diseases are also symbols and fulfillments of—often unspeakable—life courses. Beyond individuals and family, diseases are likewise powerful social symbols, metaphors of whole cultures and ages. Not all diseases become organizing metaphors, and their

bearers social cynosures (La Barre 1956). But the ones that do become for the scholar of any discipline one (among many) royal road
to the psychosocial dynamics of a society or of a historical epoch. To
come to know that disease metaphor is to uncover the medical biography of the group, its group-fantasy about itself, its images, atti-
tudes, values, assumptions, expectations, hopes, and dreads. A culture (or an age) manifests itself through those symbols that express
how and about what its members most deeply feel.

In her book, *Illness as Metaphor* (1979), novelist and critic Susan
Sontag revealed the nineteenth and twentieth centuries in new ways
to us: the nineteenth through an analysis of tuberculosis as an organizing metaphor, and the twentieth through an analysis of cancer as an
organizing metaphor. Thus disease is not only a biochemical process,
a possible fulfillment of a life course, and a projective screen for personal meanings; it can also serve as a "social text" which both society
and scholars interpret. Sontag writes that "TB was a disease in the
service of a romantic view of the world. Cancer is now in the service
of a simplistic view of the world that can turn paranoid" (p. 68). In a
review essay discussing Sontag's book, I wrote that

> The study of the language associated with TB and cancer quickly
> offer insight into the world view of that age. TB was the apothe-
> osis of beatification; cancer is the incarnation of evil. Those con-
> sumed with TB were heroic victims; with few exceptions [actor
> John Wayne as one] those consumed by cancer are stigmatized
> as the living dead.
>
> Let me take TB even further. TB fits perfectly into the ro-
> mantic age of hysteria. The victim of TB was seen as imbued
> with pure spirituality. Possessing an angelic, fragile counte-
> nance, such a person was above sensuality. At the same time, to
> have TB was to receive permission for libertinism, an indul-
> gence of the passions that purportedly was due to the illness.
> (Death is thus both fulfillment of spiritualization and restitution
> for having given into the consuming desire.) Freud's *Studies on
> Hysteria* might have been conducted in a TB sanitarium!
>
> Cancer, on the other hand, is Curse itself. It is an unending
> Orson Wellesian nightmare of foreign intrusion, unsuspected
> terror that overruns, controls, consumes, and destroys—all

with the helpless compliance of the host whose very machinery is used for self-destruction. Cancer is the Alien Other. Cancer is death sentence by pronouncement. Unmistakably, cancer is our most potent voodoo death, our most durable vessel for paranoia (1979:35).

Today I would add that AIDS has joined the ranks of disease symbols, probably even surpassing in dread that of cancer. To Americans AIDS condenses into a single image of imagined punishment for sexual pleasure, a regression from heterosexuality to an obsession with homosexuality, and the rise of a neo-puritan climate.

I have introduced the topic of disease and symbolism to help enrich the reading of *Medical Biographies*. For never is disease simply a biomedical entity in the life of an individual, family, and society. And to denude it of subjectivity and to declare that the only legitimate interpretation is mechanical or technological—this is our preeminent myth, our age's official subjectivity. Disease itself is often the outcome of hidden meanings; it certainly is attributed meanings—by oneself, one's family, one's community, one's culture—once it is diagnosed. In a brilliant paper called "Cancer and Death in the Promethean Age," Ellen Golub argues that cancer fits the self-image of our age "because it is a symbol of our desires and our abnormal expansion" (1981:727). "Cancer becomes a screen upon which we project our anxieties about our own power" (p. 728). "Cancer is, for us, a metaphor of our powers gone wild. . . . Autonomy, power, and will: these are the core of meaning with which this metaphor is 'awash'" (p. 729). The horror of cancer is the underside of our deification of technology—itself the extension of our own hubris. In *Medical Biographies*, the reader learns not only the effect of disease upon historical figures living in different times, but—with a little extra work—the symbolism of disease as well.

Dale is an engaging raconteur. His narratives should be of interest to medical historians, medical sociologists, medical anthropologists, Europeanists, Americanists, psychobiographers, family historians, and the many—professionals and laity alike—whose tincture of schadenfreude account for an interest in diseases which have done in those thought to be "larger than life." Dale's rich caselike studies also merit inclusion in medical-student, residency-training, and nurs-

ing curricula as well. With the emphasis on "the whole person," "ho-
lism," and "contextual thinking" that are at least the shibboleths—if
not actual ideals—of behavioral science-enriched medical education
since the 1960s, this book should surely have a place in bringing the
subject of medicine to life. I will do my best to find a place for it in
my own teaching of medical humanities. Experts of all kinds will
cavil over details in various chapters; and who among us does not
have a historical hero or two (or villain) he or she would have wished
had been included in Dale's medical pantheon? The book's real or
imagined flaws pale when compared with its accomplishment: a
multidisciplinary synthesis that should inspire us to broaden our
perceptions about the human experience of disease.

REFERENCES

Golub, Ellen. "Cancer and Death in the Promethean Age," *Journal of
    Popular Culture* 14 (4) (Spring 1981): 725–31.
La Barre, Weston. "Social Cynosure and Social Structure." In *Per-
    sonal Character and Cultural Milieu*, Douglas G. Haring, ed. New
    York, Syracuse University Press, 1956, pp. 535–63.
Sontag, Susan. *Illness as Metaphor*. New York, Vintage/Random
    House, 1979.
Stein, Howard F. Review essay on *Illness as Metaphor*, *The Journal of
    Psychological Anthropology* 3 (1) (Winter 1979): 33–38.
Weisman, Avery D., and Robert K. Kastenbaum. *The Psychological
    Autopsy*. New York, Human Sciences Press, 1968.

PREFACE

THIS WORK is not a study in vital statistics. Obviously both the causes of disability and the causes of death among famous persons are not different from those affecting the contemporary adult population in general. What I have tried to do is to illuminate a dark corner of legitimate biography, in a few select instances, with the light of modern medical understanding. A clearer meaning of observed symptoms, the result of an immense accumulation of necropsy and laboratory data by thousands of investigators in many lands, has made the volume possible; the eager appetite of the literate public for biographical fare, coupled with recent popular interest in medical science, has seemed to make it timely.

Throughout the book an effort has been made to avoid the jargon of medicine as far as it was possible to do so without sacrificing essential matter. Although the appeal is directed at the layman, I venture to hope that my fellow members of the medical profession may find something of interest in its pages.

The search for medical information on persons of remote times has generally ended in frustration. Only occasionally has it been possible, by picking up a few symptomatic threads here and a few more there, to weave a fabric of diagnosis. But the acquisition of necessary information was, in itself, not enough. Admittedly, without the aid and encouragement of certain able and kindly persons, completion of this volume would have been impossible. It is, therefore, in a spirit of gratitude that I acknowledge my

Medical Biographies

special indebtedness to Edward Everett Dale, research professor of history in the University of Oklahoma, for instruction in the methods of historical investigation and for his general helpfulness; to Dr. Kellogg Speed, professor of surgery in the Medical School of the University of Illinois, whose wide surgical experience and unusual academic scholarship were freely consulted; to Dr. Walter Wessels, emeritus professor of medicine in the College of Medical Evangelists and present member of the California State Board of Medical Examiners, for critical review of manuscripts and for pertinent suggestions.

Thanks are due the Package Library of the American Medical Association, Chicago; the Library of the Los Angeles County Medical Association; the Library of the Surgeon General's Office, Washington, D. C.; the Medical Library of the University of Southern California; the Los Angeles City Library; and several state, city, and private libraries for aid in obtaining indispensable material. Finally, to Mrs. Josephine Nicholson Bond and Mrs. Billie Cutright Forrester, who typed the manuscript for publication, praise for an onerous task well done.

Philip Marshall Dale, M.D.

Los Angeles, California

THE FAMOUS PERSONS

Medical Biographies

PORTRAITS

xvii

All these portraits were provided by Culver Service

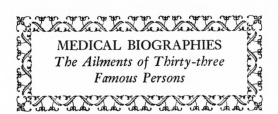

MEDICAL BIOGRAPHIES
The Ailments of Thirty-three
Famous Persons

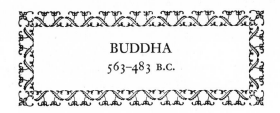

GAUTAMA, surnamed Buddha because he was held to have attained *bodhi*, or supreme knowledge, was born of noble parentage in the principality of Kapalavistau in ancient India. As a young prince he was strong, brave, and skilled in the use of weapons. He is said to have won his beautiful wife by a series of contests at arms with a number of rival chiefs.

For the first ten years of their married life the couple lived the carefree and useless existence of the idle rich. Then, reflecting on the human misery that everywhere met his eye as he drove through the city, Gautama became sober and brooding. "The world," said he, "is built on pain and its foundations are laid in agony." At about the age of thirty he abandoned his wife and child, who were amply provided for, and exchanging his princely raiment for the rags of a passing beggar, took up his abode in a cave in the wilderness. There, in primeval quiet, he evolved the system of religious philosophy which is identified with his name.

For six years he subsisted on a diet consisting chiefly of mosses, roots, seeds, and wild fruits. As a result of this fare he became greatly emaciated, and since it was deficient in proteins, he undoubtedly became very weak also. Later he returned to the conventional diet of the times, but he was always temperate with respect to both food and drink. In general, his health seems to have been good.

3

Because of his democratic ideals and the universality of his compassion, he mingled freely with all classes of society and all types of individuals. In the last few months of his life, it is told, he was lavishly entertained by a group of nobles on one occasion and on another he and his monks were treated to a splendid dinner by a famous courtesan named Ambapala who owned the grove in which the Master had been holding a sort of camp meeting. When the meal was finished, Ambapala dedicated the grove to pious uses.

Having concluded his sermons in the grove, Buddha proceeded to a near-by village to enter retreat. While at retreat he became acutely ill, but the symptoms of his sickness are not described. It is stated, however, that he shook off his illness because the time was not ripe for entering Nirvana. After recovering from illness and upon completion of retreat, he resumed his sacred peregrinations which, after three months, brought him to Pava, where he set up camp in a mango grove. The owner of the grove was a person of intermediate social status—a blacksmith named Cunda. The smith, not wishing to appear inferior to the others in his manner of honoring the worthy guest, likewise prepared a feast for Buddha and his suite. The menu was excellent, consisting of hard and soft foods, sweet rice, truffles, and another dish which was especially pleasing to the guest of honor, who asked that this food be served to him alone. The nature of the favored comestible, which was called "sukaramaddova," is in doubt, but the consensus of early writers indicates that the principal ingredient was pork.

Buddha partook freely of the sukaramaddova, but apparently felt some internal uneasiness soon thereafter, for he commanded his host to bury the uneaten portion in a deep hole in the ground, remarking that the others would not be able to digest it. Shortly he was seized with cruel pain and great weakness. He is said to have suffered a "flow of blood," presumably from the bowels. Desiring not to disturb the festivity of the occasion, he tried to conceal his suffering and called his close companion, a monk named Anandra, saying, "Let us proceed to Kusinara." The pair thanked their host and then took their leave, walking slowly along the road. As they neared the village, Buddha paused at the foot of a tree and asked the monk to fold a robe and place it on the ground. He

4

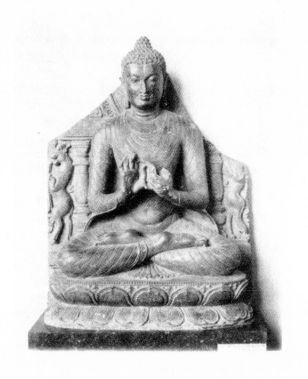

BUDDHA

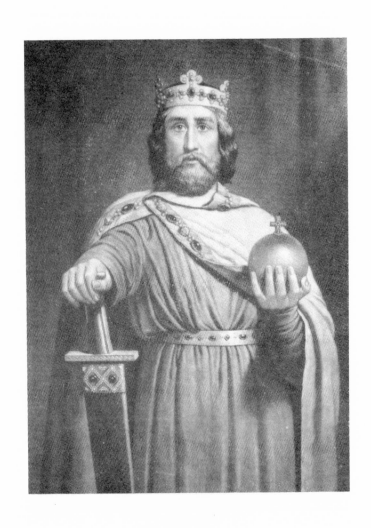

CHARLEMAGNE

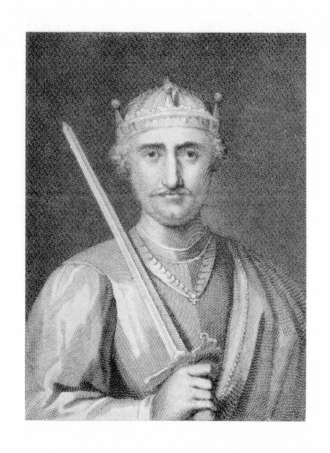

WILLIAM THE CONQUEROR

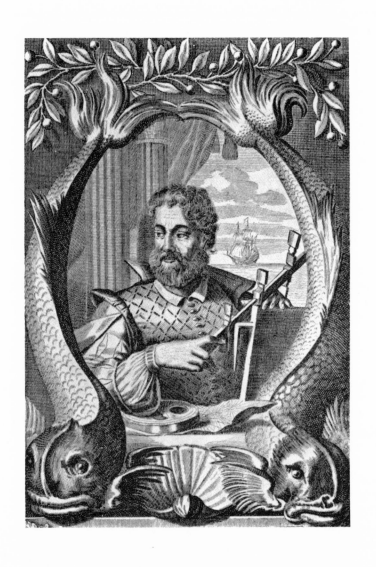

CHRISTOPHER COLUMBUS

then sat down on the robe and bade the monk fetch some water at once. So acute was his thirst that he called three times before water could be procured from the near-by river.

After drinking freely of the water brought by Anandra, he evidently felt better, for shortly he arose and walked to the river, where he bathed and drank more water. He resumed the journey, but at the outskirts of the village he was again overcome by weakness and forced to lie down on the robe as before. He lay on his right side, and as he rested he conversed freely with the villagers who had gathered about him. He evinced no sign of pain, but his increasing weakness was plain to all. Near the end he swooned and seemed to die, but his great determination revived him and he was able to make the final exhortation and promise. Then he closed his eyes and in a few moments ceased to breathe.

In essaying a diagnosis of the cause of death, we have a sequence of symptoms to guide us. First is the sudden onset of illness after partaking of a hearty meal; next is the passing of blood; third is the extreme thirst; and last is the fatal issue without, apparently, much terminal pain. This symptom complex points straight to internal hemorrhage.

Acute coronary obstruction is ruled out by the passing of blood and the extreme thirst, which are absolutely uncharacteristic of that very common cause of sudden death. Moreover, the final moments were clear and tranquil, which is rare in cases of exodus by the coronary route. Possibility of cerebral hemorrhage is excluded by absence of paralysis or immediate disturbance of intellectual function. Acute pancreatitis of the degree of severity necessary to produce death in so short a time is characterized by persistent agonizing pain, vomiting, and quick and complete collapse. Death by perforated gastric or intestinal ulcer is rarely complicated by hemorrhage and of itself does not cause death until the lapse of several days.

Granting that death resulted from internal hemorrhage, a question arises concerning the nature and location of the lesion. Since the bleeding was evidently rapid and profuse, it probably came from a deep-seated ulceration involving not only the mucous surface of the digestive tract but the deeper muscular layer as well, and as no mention is made of vomiting, we must conclude

5

that the ulcer lay below the level of the stomach. That being so, it follows that it was almost surely located in the duodenum. Carcinoma may occur anywhere in the intestinal tract and is often ulcerated. But very, very rarely is ulcerated carcinoma of the bowel the source of acute, fatal hemorrhage.

The probable sequence of events was as follows: After the ingestion of a large quantity of irritating food an attack of acute indigestion with violent, painful peristalsis ensued. A sizable artery, lying in or contiguous to an ulcer, ruptured and loosed a large quantity of blood into the intestinal tract. Most of this blood was expelled by the bowels. When the sick man lay down the bleeding stopped or was greatly slowed. But with resumption of the upright posture and muscular activity it began anew or was much accelerated. Meantime tissue fluids had been drawn into the circulatory system to dilute the blood remaining in the vessels and slow down the clotting process. When the victim lay down the second time, he obtained little or no relief. The flow persisted, though it may have accumulated in the bowel without further expulsion. Finally, loss of circulating-fluid volume combined with oxygen deficiency resulted in the stoppage of cardiac function.

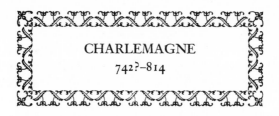

CHARLEMAGNE
742?–814

IN THE OPINION of most students of the period, Charles the Great, perhaps better known as Charlemagne, is the most imposing figure to grace the pages of Medieval history. His successes on the battlefield and his achievements as legislator and administrator have been recorded by many writers, but it has remained for a single author to give us an intimate, personal view of Charles the man.

For this human portrait of the great Frankish king, we are indebted to one Einhard, or Eginhard, as his name is sometimes written. Einhard was Charles' personal friend and secretary. The original manuscript is in Latin and the several translations, as we might expect, are at variance in a few items. In essential matters, there is no serious disagreement. It is entitled *Vita Caroli* and in the language of Hodgkin, is "one of the most precious bequests of the Middle Ages."

Since Charles was approximately thirty years of age when Einhard was born, it seems a safe assumption that the Charles with the "rather prominent belly" who was in the "habit of awakening and arising from his bed four or five times during the night" was at least well started in middle life when his secretary-biographer first entered the royal service.

In person Charles was described as "large and strong and of lofty stature," though not disproportionately tall, his height being

7

"seven times the length of his foot." Unfortunately, the length of his foot is not given and the equation has no mathematical value. Perhaps it was the intention of the biographer to stress proportion rather than size, an ideal derived from the Greeks. According to Gray, the length of the foot of the white adult male averages ten inches. Occasionally it is as little as eight inches and rarely as much as fourteen inches. As anyone may observe, tall men usually have longer feet than those of lesser height, but there are notable exceptions. Robert Fitzsimmons, one-time heavyweight boxing champion, was seventy-one inches in height, weighed 165–70 pounds in condition, and could comfortably wear a size six shoe, which means that his foot was not more than eight and one-half inches in length. The common statement that Charles was "seven feet tall' seems to be based on the assumption that his foot measured twelve inches in length. It seems likely that had he been so extremely tall, the secretary would have been less restrained in his language.

Continuing the description, "the upper part of the head was round, eyes large and animated, nose a little long, hair fair, and face laughing and merry. Thus his appearance was always stately and dignified whether he was standing or sitting, although his neck was thick and somewhat short and his belly rather prominent, but the symmetry of the rest of the body concealed these defects. His gait was firm, his whole carriage manly, and his voice clear but not so strong as his size led one to expect."

Charles had a palace near Aix-la-Chapelle where he greatly enjoyed bathing in the warm springs. Sometimes he would have as many as a hundred fellow bathers in the water with him, and yet not one of them, it is said, could outswim the King.

He was temperate in his eating and particularly so in his drinking. His meals consisted of four courses, not counting the roast venison of which he was fonder than of any other dish. "He abominated drunkenness" and was so temperate that he rarely had more than three cups of wine or other sorts of drink in the course of a meal. In summer he would eat some fruit after the midday meal and drink a cup of wine which, presumably, was not added to the three customarily taken with the meal. Then he would take off his shoes and have a good nap of two or three hours' duration.

His marital record reads like a war casualty list. His first marriage, to a daughter of Desiderius, he repudiated after one year. After her came three wives in fatal succession. What caused their deaths is not known. His second wife left three sons and three daughters; his third wife departed this life after bearing two daughters. He had no children by either his first or his fourth wife. Finding himself a widower for the fourth time, Charles apparently became discouraged with marriage and put his trust in concubines, of which some say he had four and some say a large number. It is known that he had five children by four concubines. It is possible that others, being childless, escaped identification.

For many years Charles was accustomed to get up several times nightly probably because of an irritable bladder due to prostatism. Otherwise his health had always been good until the age of sixty-eight. Then he began to have fevers with increasing frequency. These he was accustomed to control by fasting. Toward the last he limped a little on one foot. What caused his bouts of fever is a matter for conjecture. It may well be that they were due to an infection of the genito-urinary tract, a common occurrence in men with hypertrophied prostates, and that abstinence from irritating food and drink improved his bladder function and ameliorated the unpleasant symptoms. At all times "he consulted his own inclinations" and disdained the advice of the physicians, "who were almost hateful to him" because they wanted him to give up roasts and eat boiled meat instead.

Early in his decline observant persons saw many portents of Charles' approaching doom. For one thing, there were frequent eclipses of both the sun and moon, and at one time a black spot was visible on the sun for a space of seven days. But there were plenty of premonitions close at hand. The gallery between the basilica and the palace at Aix-la-Chapelle suddenly crashed to earth on Ascension Day; the wooden bridge which Charles had built across the Rhine at Mayence was consumed by an accidental fire; a large ball of fire once swished across the sky frightening Charles' steed, which shied and threw the rider heavily to the ground; and whenever the King entered a building, a continuous crackling noise ensued. Perhaps the most sinister omen of all was given when the gilded ball on the roof of the basilica was struck by a bolt of

9

lightning and hurled on to the adjacent roof of the bishop's house. Despite the obvious significance of all these manifestations, Charles seemed to have no foreboding of evil; on the contrary, he continued to labor with undiminished zeal for the advancement of learning and religion throughout the wide expanses of his kingdom.

In the autumn of 813, despite his weakening condition, the King engaged in a strenuous and protracted hunt as had been his custom each fall for many years, and in November he returned to the palace for the winter. In the month of January, however, he was seized with a high fever which he endeavored to cure by fasting—a remedy he had employed successfully against other attacks of fever. But this one seemed to be different. It was more resistant, and "besides the fever he suffered from a pain in the side which the Greeks call 'pleurisy.' " Nevertheless, he continued to fast, keeping up his strength only by "draughts" taken at long intervals. He failed, however, to outlast his sickness. On the morning of the seventh day after he had taken to his bed, he died quietly, as becomes a man of strong intellect, great dignity, and stout spirit.

Sudden high fever, pleurisy, and exodus at the end of one week constitute a symptomatic triad characteristic of lobar pneumonia. In common with other acute respiratory-tract infections, pneumonia is especially prone to occur in the winter months. Almost surely the great warrior-king was struck down by that once-dread disease which Osler in his time aptly termed "Captain of the Men of Death."

So deep was the impress which the personality of Charles had made upon the minds of men that it was impossible for them to believe he was dead. Only Nature, twitching and shuddering at the prospect of his passing, became quickly tranquil and resumed the even tenor of her way.

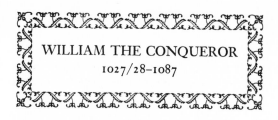

WILLIAM THE CONQUEROR
1027/28–1087

ABOUT THE YEAR 1026, Robert, young count of the Hiesmais and son of Duke Richard, was approaching his capital of Falaise when he spied Arlette, daughter of a local tanner, on the bank of a near-by stream. According to one account, the young woman was washing linen; according to another, she was disporting herself in the dance. It is possible, of course, that the contradiction is more apparent than real. Youth being what it is, which presumably is what it was even in the dull days of medievalism, Arlette may have decided merely to take a little time out from her wash to frisk off an exuberance of animal spirits. And then again, she may have seen the count first.

Whatever the facts, it is safe to assume that some livelier emotion than a mere admiration for her domesticity impelled the count to ride up to the girl, seize her, and carry her off to his castle where, without benefit of clergy, she served him quite as faithfully and as variously as a wife might have done up to the day of his death seven or eight years later. It was by way of this episode that William the Bastard was given to the world. And it was in appreciation of it that, when in his mature years the Duke confronted the defenses of Alençon, the taunt, "hides for the tanner," which the jeering enemy hurled at him, angered him far more than did the shower of missiles which accompanied the gibe.

In the years of his adolescence William had a parlous time of it. His father, Duke Robert, died while returning from a holy pilgrimage in the year 1035, and the news of his death immediately plunged the country into a state of wildest anarchy. Young Duke William was kept in hiding for a dozen years, at the end of which period he emerged to take revenge on his enemies. Although he was not over twenty years of age at this time, he was said to have had both the appearance and the judgment of a much older and more experienced warrior. In the ripeness of his manhood he was of medium height with rather a long neck linking a thick, powerful body with a large head, bald in front and hair closely cropped. He was so strong of arm that with his horse at full gallop he could draw a bow that defied the exertions of any other man with his feet firmly planted on solid ground. In his personal life he was so apathetic in his behavior toward likely women that, in an age of licentiousness, he was commonly believed to be impotent. He was inordinately fond of hunting and, according to an old chronicle, "he loved the tall deer as if he were their father."

About the year 1063, William was seized by a severe illness that brought him to the slippery brink of death. At a time when illness was regarded as either a visitation of divine wrath or a machination of the devil, depending on the conscience of the victim and the preferences of those who knew him, little attention was paid to symptoms. All we know about this illness is contained in a quotation from Stinton, "So sore bestead was he that he was laid on the ground as one about to die, and in his extreme need he gave the reliquary which accompanied him on his progress, to the Church of St. Mary of Constances." Since he was laid on the ground, we may suppose that his illness had a sudden and violent onset; we can be certain only that he recovered. Shortly after the Battle of Hastings, the army was hit by an epidemic of dysentery, and anon William was stricken by an acute illness, probably the same that had the army on its haunches. He was laid up for several weeks and the mark of his illness was upon him for several more.

It usually happens that the heavy-bodied youth, quick and active though he may be, becomes a corpulent and unwieldly man at middle age. It was so with William, and so it came about that in the summer of 1087 he journeyed to Rouen for a course of medicine to relieve his obesity—the thin man within him was crying for release. Wherefore, Philip of France, having heard of the Conqueror's womanish recourse, remarked that the "fat man" was "lying in," implicitly with child. The outraged William, pursuing the theme of Philip's comment, replied that he would do his churching in Paris and burn a thousand candles, it being a custom of the times that a woman fresh from childbed would burn a candle in the church for each babe. Then, with fire in his eye, the fat one mounted his charger, rallied his army to his side, and roared into the French Vexin, bent first on retaliation against the garrison at Mantes for incursions into his territory. The city was quickly captured, sacked, and burned. But he did not get to Paris. As William was riding among the smoldering ruins of stricken Mantes, his horse is believed to have stepped into a bed of embers which caused the animal to plunge and throw the rider violently against the pommel of the saddle. It was immediately obvious that he had suffered a serious internal injury.

The Conqueror was carried to Rouen, where he lay for nearly a month tortured by pain, and tormented by the heat, flies, and the innumerable noises of the city. He bade his attendants carry him to St. Gervaise, which stands on a hill to the west of the town, where he was lodged in the priory. There, in monastic quiet, he reflected upon his sinful past, and in agony of spirit as much as of body he begged Heaven and earth for forgiveness of the excesses of his despotism and gave voluminous directions for reparations to be made to the victims of his harshness. He even consented to the release from prison of his half-brother, Odo, though he foretold that liberty for the villain would mean ruin and death for many innocent persons. To make the record complete, he also related the story of his life to his sons, William and Henry, and to his physician as well as to the bishops, abbots, and all who had come to witness the demise of their lord and were in a mood to listen.

On the night of September 8–9, the severity of his pain having somewhat abated, he slept peacefully until daybreak. Then, as the bells of St. Mary's Church tolled for primes, he awoke, folded his hands in prayer, and forthwith expired. His friends, being assured that William was dead and recalling the state of anarchy which had followed upon announcement of the death of Duke Robert fifty-two years before, fled to their homes leaving

13

the body in the care of attendants. By the time the clergy had roused and come to the death chamber, the body had been stripped, the room plundered, and the place deserted.

The archbishop directed that the corpse should be carried to the church which William had founded at Caen many years before, but no man of proper rank could be found to accompany it. Finally, however, a minor knight named Herlwin was chosen for the honor. As the cortege neared the city and a procession of clergy and townsfolk was coming forth to join it, a burst of flame was seen arising from the town. A live fire being more important, in the circumstances, than a dead king, the citizens rushed back to the conflagration, leaving only a few faithful monks to carry the body to their quarters outside the walls of the city.

During the funeral services, which were conducted by a bishop of Evreaux in the presence of the prelates of the Norman church, one of the congregation named Ascelin stamped forward and loudly declared that the spot where the grave had been prepared was once the courtyard of his father's home and that the same had been forcibly and unjustly seized by the dead man for the foundation of his abbey. Ascelin would listen to reason only if it was accompanied by the tinkle of silver. So, after a short but unseemly interruption, the claim was adjudicated, a first payment was made to the claimant, and the services resumed. When the body was lifted from the bier and transferred to the newly made sarcophagus, it was discovered that the fit was a little on the snug side. Pressure was applied with explosive effect. Apparently William was harboring a large abscess within his abdomen as a result of his injury, which purulent accumulation had been augmented by post-mortem decay. The abdominal wall, already near the bursting point, was unable to withstand further pressure. As the stench was wafted through the chapel the mourners, hands to noses, made for the door in panicky haste. The burial party clapped the lid on the coffin as well as the exigencies of the situation would permit and interment was hastily concluded.

The Conqueror's bones were allowed to moulder peacefully until the year 1562 when the Hugenots, in futile spitefulness, dug them up and strewed them about the place.

The immediate cause of William's death appears to have been

a slowly spreading abscess within his abdominal cavity. It seems probable that, as a result of the accident already described, there was an injury to the lower bowel of such nature and severity as to permit some degree of leakage of intestinal contents into the peritoneal cavity. The fact that acute, spreading peritonitis and death did not ensue within a few days after the injury was sustained is significant. It indicates that the leakage was small in amount and possibly of delayed occurrence, permitting a "walling-off" reaction to take place between peritoneal surfaces adjacent to the wound in the bowel. For six weeks the walled-in pus slowly increased in quantity, pushing back protective barriers until septic absorption resulted in death. If, as could have happened, the abscess had burrowed its way through the abdominal wall before death instead of after that event, the Conqueror might have gone on to an end better befitting the rampageous warrior that he was. In that case his obsequies might have been more imposing, though they could hardly have been more memorable.

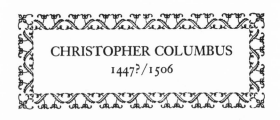

IT IS AN OLD OBSERVATION that the abode of greatness commonly presents an unimposing or even shabby exterior. In the case of Christopher Columbus, although an authentic portrait is lacking, there is good reason to believe his physical attributes were in keeping with the heroic character of the man. Testimony from many sources reveals that the discoverer of America was tall, strongly built, and of commanding presence. He had a ruddy complexion with a scattering of freckles, an aquiline nose, gray eyes, and light reddish hair. He is said to have been temperate in his eating and drinking, deeply religious, and puritanical in his private life.

His heredity was favorable. His father lived to "an extreme age" and his mother was apparently about seventy at the time of her death. Both parents were of healthy, hearty Ligurian peasant stock. The son, Christopher, was the eldest of five children who lived to maturity. He went to sea at an early age but was about forty-five when on Friday, August 3, 1492, he sailed westward from the little port of *Palos de la Frontera,* Spain, to inaugurate an epoch of maritime discovery. He was gone 225 days and during the entire period seems to have suffered no ailment other than a spell of sore eyes, believed to have been caused by prolonged looking against the bright sun-rays as he gazed hopefully toward the western horizon.

On the Second Voyage, he sailed from Cádiz on September 25, 1493, and reached San Domingo on November 27. He spent the winter on that island, putting to sea again on April 24, 1494, to discover Jamaica, Hispaniola, and the islets of Beata, Saona, and Mona. On November 25, he went into a state of collapse thought to have been the result of prolonged anxiety and loss of sleep. "He lay in a stupor, knowing little, remembering nothing, his eyes dim and vitality oozing until the little fleet sorrowfully but gladly returned to the Harbor of Isabella," San Domingo, on September 29. For nearly five months he was prostrate, for several weeks of which he lay muttering in a low delirium, totally unable to feed or care for himself. De Ybarra believes that the Admiral had typhus, typhoid, or relapsing fever—most likely typhus. During this illness he was cared for by Dr. Diego Alvarez Chanca, whose extra-professional notes on the voyage are of singular interest and value.

As he recovered from his illness, Columbus found it advisable to take account of the health of his men. A "scourge" had incapacitated so many of the fleet's personnel that the Admiral at one time "determined to leave the search for the mines until he had first despatched the ships which were to return to Spain on account of the great sickness which had prevailed among the men." Morison, quoting Aguado, states: "Almost everyone in Isabella was sick or discontented and eager to go home." The sickness may have been syphilis, which, in the opinion of most syphilographers, is of New World origin and was carried to the Old World by sailors returning from the Second Voyage. Early in March, 1496, the fleet began its homeward trip, arriving on June 11. The stock of provisions had run so low that starvation threatened, and the thirty to forty Indian captives who were being taken to Spain barely escaped the galley pots.

On the Third Voyage, Columbus had a fleet of six ships and two hundred men in addition to the crews. They left the tiny seaport town of Barrameda on May 30, 1498. In the last days of June, according to Irving, as Columbus "advanced within the tropics the change of climate and the close, sultry weather brought on a severe attack of gout followed by a violent fever." This does not sound like gout. The etiology is all wrong and a violent fever has no place in the symptomatology of gout. But in the days of

17

both Columbus and Irving the term "gout" was wont to be applied by laymen and doctors alike to any type of arthritis. Descriptions of this attack and the subsequent history of his case indicate strongly that the Admiral actually had rheumatic fever. During August "he suffered a great deal from gout and ophthalmia [eye inflammation]," says Navarette. It is pertinent to remark here that inflammation of one or both eyes frequently occurs in the course of rheumatic fever. There is no good evidence, it may be added, to indicate that Columbus ever had syphilis, though the incidence of the disease among his men was probably very high.

Upon his arrival at Isabella on August 30, 1500, the Admiral was immediately put in irons and cast into prison by Francisco de Bobadilla, who had been commissioned by Ferdinand and Isabella to go out to Hispaniola and restore order in that rebellious colony. To the great disadvantage of Columbus, his enemies had got to Bobadilla first and filled the Commissioner's ears with complaints and lies. While in prison, the unfortunate Admiral was again stricken with fever, and aching, swollen joints. Early in October he was placed aboard a vessel bound for Spain. The captain of the returning caravel offered to remove the shackles now that escape was impossible, but the proud-spirited prisoner rejected the offer, saying that he was in irons by orders of their Majesties and he would so remain until they ordered his release. Luckily the passage was calm, fair, and expeditious, and Alonzo de Villejo, who was his keeper, became also his devoted servant. On the way home Columbus wrote a long and pathetic letter to Donna Juana de la Torre, nurse of Prince Juan and a person in high favor with the Queen. This letter bore evidence of a badly overwrought nervous system. Undoubtedly it was read by Isabella, which was as Columbus had designed. His property rights, which had been automatically suspended upon his arrest and imprisonment, were eventually restored, but his status as colonizer was lost. Thereafter he was rated merely explorer and discoverer.

During the seventeen months intervening between his arrival from the Third Voyage and his departure on the Fourth, no mention is made of his "gout" or any other ailment. Alternate periods of activity and quiescence, however, are quite as characteristic of rheumatic arthritis as of true gout.

On May 11, 1502, the fleet of four caravels and 135 men sailed out of Cádiz on the Admiral's fourth and last voyage to the Western world. He did not attempt to command *La Capitana* (the flag caravel) but, suggests Morison, "perhaps because of his advancing age and precarious health," assigned this responsibility to his "former shipmate and loyal servant," Diego Tristan. The expedition was a complete failure. All the ships were lost, the Admiral's arthritis had him down much of the time, and when he was rescued finally and brought back to Barrameda, he was too sick to go to court to render an account of the voyage. Early in May, 1505, however, he managed to go to court to "plead for his rights," King Ferdinand having reneged on some of his most alluring promises. But Isabella had died the year before and there was no one to lend a sympathetic ear to the entreaties of the unhappy petitioner.

There can be no doubt that the Royal Court regarded the Admiral as a great nuisance. For nearly two years his sole activity between sick spells was the business of pestering Ferdinand with requests for adjustment of what were technically rightful claims. When the Royal Court was moved to Valladolid, Columbus followed painfully on mule-back. In that city he was given bed and board by a kindly fellow sailor named Gil García. In Valladolid, the Admiral's condition grew steadily worse. First his legs and then his belly swelled hideously and he could not lie flat in bed. He was in the terminal stage of rheumatic heart disease.

On Ascension Day, May 20, 1506, death, as it must to all men, came to Christopher Columbus.

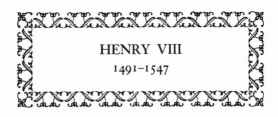

HENRY VIII
1491-1547

HENRY VII, King of England, had a cough. He had coughed from the time he was thirty years old, and that was in 1487, thirteen years ago—coughed a little more each year and grown a little thinner and paler, too. He had weak lungs, the doctors said, and should work less and sleep more. But Henry was a dynast, the first of the House of Tudor, and there was work to be done. He was also a miser and misers do not die easily. They cling tenaciously to anything they esteem, whether it is gold or life. So Henry worked and hoarded—and coughed.

In 1486, Henry's queen had borne a son. He was the first male child and therefore the heir apparent. But he was a puny baby, poorly developed and unpromising in appearance. Consequently, when in 1491, the dutiful queen yielded another son, a robust, lusty-lunged moppet, the king was happy. It was comforting to feel that "just in case . . . ." The infant was named Henry.

It was hoped that the first son, Prince Arthur, would outgrow his weakness, but as he grew older it seemed to center in his chest. The old king had provided the soil and the seed too. Arthur was tuberculous.

Ferdinand and Isabella of Spain had a daughter who was a little more than a year older than Arthur. Ferdinand was afraid of France. Henry also was afraid of France. If a marriage could be arranged between Catherine and Arthur, it would automatically ally Spain and England. Henry thought that would be good for

England and hoped Ferdinand would consider it good for Spain. But England was small and the seat on the Tudor throne precarious; Ferdinand needed a bit of convincing. So Henry dispatched Bishop Fox to Spain, not to argue Arthur's intrinsic worth as a son-in-law, for that would be nothing, but to point out to the Spanish rulers how the match would accrue to the benefit of Spain. The bishop was well chosen. He made a plausible case of it and the wedding was duly solemnized with appropriate pomp and circumstance.

The young couple were installed at Ludlow Court. For five months they rehearsed the regal role. Then one day Arthur cried out in pain, fell to the floor, and was carried to the princely chamber by shaken and pale-faced courtiers. The morbid pulmonary process, probably in the form of a caseous focus beneath the pulmonary pleura, had broken through the cover of the lung into the pleural space permitting air to enter between the lung and the chest wall. The result was pneumothorax—collapse of the lung, displacement of the heart and great vessels, and terrific shock. A few days later Arthur was dead, and Catherine, the young widow, had not become Queen of England. Her mission had failed and her trading value was seriously impaired. True, there was young Henry, the picture of health and juvenile vigor. The six years difference in their ages was on the wrong side, but it would grow relatively less as time went on. The situation might be patched up, at that. But, on the other hand, there was Leviticus, in which is written, "And if a man shall take his brother's wife, it is impurity. He hath uncovered his brother's nakedness. They shall be childless." The prospect of a childless marriage was chilling to the Tudor dynasts. But had Catherine actually been Arthur's wife? There was much secret confabulation between the Spanish lady in waiting, the Spanish chamberlain, and the Spanish confessor. If Catherine were proved not a virgin, it would be an international calamity with Spain on the heavy end. Catherine simply had to be a virgin. Donna Elvira, Catherine's lady, could make the necessary and fateful examination with the least embarrassment to Catherine. It was so arranged. The Donna emerged from the bed chamber exultant. "As intact as the day she left her mother's womb" was the impartial verdict. Whereupon the Spanish contingent whooped with joy.

21

There was, however, a disquieting rumor on the English side. It was told among the courtiers and attested to by a number of noblemen that the first words the young prince had uttered the morning after the wedding were, "My masters, marriage is a thirsty pastime." And when a cup of hot wine had passed through the curtain to the boy, he smiled at the servitor and announced, on a note of triumph, "Last night I was in Spain." Whether the words were or were not uttered, they must rank among the most disturbing ever imputed to the tongue of man.

With the news that Catherine had become a widow, her mother, Isabella, took command and lost no time in putting pressure on Henry to betroth his remaining son to the young widow. France was attacking Perpignan and the case was urgent. Pope Alexander, at Isabella's solicitation, issued a dispensation implying that the marriage *had* been consummated. The dispensation was intended to erase the whole question. It was supposed to have all the moral and political value of an intact virginity. Thus, on the eve of his twelfth birthday, Henry, Prince of Wales, was betrothed to Catherine of Aragon, aged eighteen.

In 1504, three years after the betrothal, Isabella died and the fortunes of Ferdinand sank to the level of desperation. King Henry had no interest in a daughter-in-law whose dowry had been only half-paid or in an ally who had no army with which to help in case of war. Poor Catherine was left to shift for herself, and it was generally accepted that the marriage engagement of Prince Henry to Catherine was no longer binding.

Meantime, King Henry had lost his consort and was marketing for a bride. He was bald, toothless, stooped, and asthmatic—and he coughed with every other breath. No woman in her right mind would have him. Apparently that was Henry's conclusion, too, for he next selected as the object of his overtures the mad Juana, daughter of Ferdinand and Isabella and relict of Philip, Archduke of Austria. She could bring Castile to him, and even if she was insane, she might bear a healthy child or two. But Juana had a certain unpalatable peculiarity; she insisted on taking with her, wherever she went, the corpse of her beloved Philip.

On Ferdinand's advice Henry suspended his suit until the Pope should persuade Juana to make a conventional disposal of the remains. Soon, however, the specter of approaching death turned Henry's mind away from matrimonial reveries. He resisted his malady with characteristic stubbornness, but the tubercule bacillus is a master strategist of siege and the time was ripe for the final assault. Even as Henry staggered and weaved about the royal household, Ferdinand, whose luck had taken an auspicious turn, bluntly wrote the stricken monarch that young Henry would be married to Catherine or a Spanish army would move against England.

The dying king, not wishing to leave a heritage of war to his son, called the lad to the deathbed and exacted a promise of marriage with Catherine of Aragon. On April 21, 1509, the old king coughed his last and cries of "Long live Henry VIII!" echoed along the winding streets and lanes of London Town.

The new king was not of his father's desiccated fiber. He was of the maternal line and in particular resembled his grandfather, the gay, charming, and stately Edward IV. Henry VIII was a huge fellow even at eighteeen. He was active, tremendously strong, fond of hunting, jousting, and wrestling, and temperate by the standards of contemporary royalty. In modern times in different circumstances he might very well be king of a college gridiron and a vision to set co-ed hearts aflutter. With his reddish hair, glowing complexion, and graceful carriage, he was by all odds the handsomest potentate of his time. On the cerebral side, he was the delight of his tutors. He applied himself assiduously, learned to speak Latin and French with correctness and facility, and became well versed in the traditions of English royalty and the Catholic church. Moreover, he was diligently observant of the prescribed religious forms and ceremonials.

The wedding in June was secret, possibly out of respect for the departed king. For Catherine it was nonetheless an occasion for the greatest joy and satisfaction. It was her entrance into the promised land.

The House of Tudor was a newcomer on the stage of history and the dynastic role demanded masculine strength and dignity. Henry must have a male heir. Catherine knew her part and played it to the best of her ability. Within a few months she was able to tell Henry that she was with child. It was joyful news but the end was sad and ignominious. The child, a female, was born dead. Early the next year her own and Henry's joy knew no bounds when she gave birth to a son. He was a plump and healthy-looking child, but he began to waste and died at seven weeks. So continued a series of birth disasters fraught with the most portentous domestic and political consequences. A third pregnancy was lost, probably about the sixth month, and a fourth at or near term. The fifth pregnancy yielded a daughter, Mary. She lived to rule England and was called "Bloody Mary" with better discrimination than Englishmen generally exercise in the application of the adjective. In 1517 there were two miscarriages and in 1518, as a final mockery, a stillborn son. Catherine had been pregnant eight times in nine years. Truly she *had* tried.

What are the medical significations of these many miscarriages and stillbirths? It is maddening to be forced to speculate when a few laboratory tests well known to modern medicine could clear the diagnostic skies like magic. Few situations could better emphasize the value of present-day laboratory methods in the diagnosis of disease.

Of the three possible causes of Catherine's fruitless travail, namely, habitual abortion, Rh negativity, and syphilis, the last looms as far and away the most likely one. Habitual abortion occurs consistently in the earlier months of pregnancy. Rh negativity, a condition in which the Rh-negative mother's blood develops a substance destructive of her own Rh-positive child's blood, seems unlikely, not impossible. In Rh negativity, the first child is usually born alive and healthy. Subsequent pregnancies, especially after the second, are likely to result in babies which are either stillborn or prone to die soon after being born. Mary's survival could be explained by the assumption that she and her mother were both Rh negative. But Mary was a puny child who, even in her girlhood, looked old, had defective vision, and a cranial conformation rather typical for congenital syphilis. She died of cerebral thrombosis, a clot formation in one or more of the blood vessels of the brain, at the age of forty-two, which is earlier than usual for death from that cause. While the birth pattern is not perfectly typical for syphilis, in that the later pregnancies did not result in living children, nevertheless available medical evidence weighs heavily in favor of syphilis as the correct explanation for the procreative frustrations of Henry and Catherine. The natural question is: When and how did Catherine become infected?

Some writers have conjectured that Henry acquired his syphilis in 1514 while he was in France at the head of a punitive expedition against Louis XII, who had incurred the British King's pious displeasure by defying Pope Julius. Henry had gone to France in the spring of the year, returning in October just a few weeks after Catherine's third parturient disaster. Soon he became mysteriously ill. "The King of England," runs one report, "has had the fever and his physicians were afraid it would turn into pustules called the smallpox." "Henry of England," runs another report, "has a fever. His physicians were afraid for his life but it ended in smallpox." Whatever the disease, it was believed to have been contracted in France and evidently there were skin manifestations. After about four months' seclusion, his majesty was declared fully recovered and "fierce against France."

The description does well enough for the skin manifestations of the secondary stage of syphilis. But Catherine had lost three babies in succession before Henry's illness appeared. Henry was thought to have had smallpox in his childhood and, moreover, syphilis is almost never appreciably febrile. It is extremely unlikely that the royal ailment was syphilis and it is doubtful if it was smallpox. A guess is that it was pustular dermatitis resulting from filthy clothing and body lice, though it could have been any one of several disorders classed as skin diseases and characterized by macular or papular eruptions and some degree of fever.

The possibility that Catherine was syphilitic prior to her marriage to Henry seems very remote, but the stern mandates of diagnostic procedure demand its consideration. Congenital syphilis is out of the question for the reasons that the disease was probably unknown in Europe at the time of her birth and the marital and family records of Ferdinand and Isabella are completely negative as far as evidence of it are concerned. Catherine, therefore, acquired her syphilis.

The diagnosis of disease is frequently a cynical business. Abundant experience with the human animal has shown that, particularly in the case of ailments related to personal morality, small reliance can be placed on piety and the solemn word. Normal-minded persons prefer to speak the truth at all times. They may be deterred, however, by a sense of shame or a desire to protect their own or someone else's interests. For example, though Catherine is reputed to have said that her marriage to Arthur was never consummated, in the conventional use of that word, few students of history believe she was virginal when she was married to Henry. On the other hand, even fewer believe that she was unchaste at any time. We must, however, hear the evidence.

Hume and others have made much of Catherine's devotion to her Spanish confessor, Friar Diego Fernández, during the days of her youthful widowhood. They point to the great influence the Friar undoubtedly wielded over Catherine and picture him as an immoral monster who could not have failed to turn that influence to his own wicked purposes. It is true that Henry, not long after his marriage to Catherine, called in the priest, denounced him for a fornicator, and sent him back to Spain. The fact that no accusation was lodged against Catherine indicates strongly that Henry harbored no suspicion whatever with respect to her conduct with the Friar. The current opinion was that the Spanish father knew too much about certain of Henry's extramarital affairs for Henry's peace of mind. So Henry, fearing derogatory publicity, decided to strike the first blow by reversing the charge—a little tactic, incidentally, not unknown to modern international diplomacy. Moreover, it seems likely that a woman with Catherine's remarkable fertility could not, in those times, have maintained relations with a healthy male without becoming pregnant. The logical conclusion is that despite his apparently perfect health and extraordinary strength and endurance, Henry was syphilitic from the days of his adolescence and had infected Catherine with the disease promptly after their marriage. The possibility that the puny, tuberculous Prince Arthur might have given Catherine her syphilis cannot, of course, be absolutely ruled out.

Henry had but recovered from his "smallpox," it is related, when a message arrived from Louis conveying positive proof that Ferdinand of Spain, Henry's father-in-law, with the collusion of Maximilian of Austria, had signed a secret truce with the King of France. It is alleged that when Henry was apprised of the deception, the impact of the astounding news changed his character completely. From then on, he grew progressively more suspicious of those about him, more vengeful, and more brutal in his punishment of any who seemed to oppose him in even the smallest matters. Along with his growing cynicism, it is related, was an increasing belief in his own infallibility and his importance in God's scheme of things. It seems probable that such changes as occurred in Henry's attitude and behavior were the normal reactions of a man who finds himself deceived by those in whom he reposed the greatest confidence and so resolves to be his own counselor. It is unlikely that they were due to syphilis of the central nervous system. His exaltation of the ego was a mere expression of independence. Subsequent events indicate that this is so. At any rate, there seems little sense in imputing to disease those grandiose ideas which, in the case of King Henry VIII, contained the substance of accomplished fact.

In 1515, it was revealed that Henry had a leg ulcer. This ulcer in a man hardly twenty-five years of age and extremely active in jousting, wrestling, and other rough sports was probably of traumatic origin. Anyhow, it was to plague him the rest of his life with its exacerbations of acute inflammation and the demand for daily attention. Failure to heal was, no doubt, the result of continued physical activity combined with lowered healing power due to syphilis. The doctors having demonstrated their inability to cure the ulcer, the patient took matters into his own hands. He made an excursion into the field of medicine, from which he emerged triumphant with a nostrum known the country over as the "King's Plaster" and "verrie goode against sores on the legs and the lykes." The ingredient believed to be most important was ground pearls. Henry treated the leg of his friend, Will Compton, who was similarly afflicted, but whether through instincts of commiseration or of experimentation is not clear. At any rate the plaster failed to heal Compton's leg.

In 1519 word came to Catherine that her husband had at last achieved a male heir. For two years Henry had engaged in an amour with one Elizabeth Blount, now nineteen years of age and one-time maid in waiting to her "serene Majesty." Young Bessie had, at the proper time, been sent to a priory and there Henry's

27

son was born. He was named Henry Fitzroy and taken from his mother to be reared in quasi-royal privacy. Later he was brought to court and given the noble rating of Duke of Richmond. Elizabeth Blount was a complaisant creature and made no outcry when her baby was taken from her nor yet when Henry switched his attentions to Mary Boleyn, elder sister of the better-known Anne.

It is of medical interest that despite the chronicity of his ailments, Henry went to France in 1520 on his famous Cloth of Gold good-will mission and played a leading role in the athletic activities of the occasion. He was angered and chagrined, it is true, when in a sudden friendly scuffle with Frances I, king of France, good King Hal, the wrestler, was rudely dumped on his royal posterior. But he later won the plaudits of the onlookers when he knocked his opponent spinning in the jousts, rode a horse till the animal fell dead, and beat every other contender at archery.

Early in 1522, Henry began to suffer qualms of conscience. Catherine had failed to yield an heir, because of God's displeasure with the marriage. Henry was being punished for taking his sister-in-law to wife. In this mood he carried on, fighting a little with France, profiting by the victories of Charles of Spain, keeping an open eye for pretenders, burning heretics, and meditating the future for the House of Tudor. Four years of accumulated despair and self-reproach, however, brought matters to the breaking point. The break was coincidental with the advent of a fascinating young Irish girl named Anne Boleyn into Henry's court. Anne was nineteen years of age and, like Elizabeth Blount, was one of the queen's maids in waiting. Henry had sought her out and she had responded to his advances. But she permitted him to go only so far and no farther. She steadfastly refused to become his mistress. She would be his queen or nothing. Henry was unaccustomed to being refused. Anne's calculated stubbornness threw him into a frenzy of desire and completely changed the course of English history. It marked the beginning of Henry's war with the Roman Catholic church and led to his secret marriage to Anne in 1533, the divorce of Catherine by English authority a few months later, and the establishment of the Church of England.

In the summer of 1528 the "sweating sickness," later known as miliary fever, struck London. The epidemic was widespread and deadly. Henry was in a panic of fear, but he seems to have escaped the disease. Anne was stricken but recovered quickly, and her survival was accepted by both as a token of Heaven's indulgence to their amour. Henry returned to the quest with augmented zeal.

In September, 1533, Anne gave birth to a daughter. The child was conceived out of wedlock, but that fact implies no relaxation of Anne's determination, for Henry had long before broken with Catherine and divorce proceedings were within inches of their goal. The infant was ill received, but she lived to be the brilliant and eccentric Queen Elizabeth who ruled England for forty-five years and died at the age of seventy.

The year following the birth of Elizabeth, Anne miscarried at four months. The accident was blamed on the emotional upset incident to a violent quarrel with the King over his attention to one of the ladies of the court. On January 29, 1536, last rites were held for Catherine, who had died of a heart ailment at the age of fifty. Anne had long desired Catherine's death, but she could not exult, for on that same day she, Queen Anne, destitute of both her husband's presence and his affection, gave birth to a dead son. Gone now was her last chance for a reconciliation with Henry. On April 18 of that year she was sent to the executioner's block on a trumped-up charge of adultery and incest. Among the spectators at the beheading was the seventeen-year-old Duke of Richmond, Henry's son by Elizabeth Blount. The young Duke, who was "tysique," began coughing up blood soon after leaving the scene and six weeks later was dead as had died his grandfather, Henry VII, and his uncle, Prince Arthur, of pulmonary tuberculosis.

Anne's miscarriages do not prove that she was syphilitic. Henry's infection had long ago ceased to be contagious, and Elizabeth, the known daughter of Anne, showed none of the stigmata of the disease. The miscarriages may have been due to emotional causes or to Rh negativity. There is a colorable theory that Elizabeth was not Henry's child; that Anne, knowing her husband's feeble procreative power, decided to seek elsewhere for the son so necessary to her security in the royal favor. The conclusion seems warranted that at least up to the time of Elizabeth's birth, Anne was untainted by syphilis.

The day following Anne's execution Henry was married to Jane Seymour, who, like Bessie Blount and Anne Boleyn, had been one of Catherine's maids in waiting but who, unlike either Bess or Anne, was a gentlewoman. In October, 1537, Jane gave birth to a son. Nine days later she was dead of childbed fever (puerperal sepsis). The infant was not vigorous, but he lived to become Edward VI and, through a regency, to rule England for six years. He was mysteriously afflicted. It is said that he had a skin eruption and that his fingers and toes dropped off. This might result from leprosy, ergot poisoning, Raynaud's vaso-spasm, or peripheral vascular disease associated with typhus, malaria, scarlet fever, syphilis, and other diseases. He died at the age of fifteen.

After three lonely years as a widower, Henry found himself betrothed to a picture bride, Anne of Cleves. Thomas Cromwell, who had succeeded Cardinal Wolsey as Henry's minister, arranged the marriage on purely political grounds. A highly idealized portrait of the new Anne had been utilized by Cromwell to arouse Henry's interest. When his Majesty laid eyes on his fiancée, he was aghast. He could not abrogate the marriage contract, but he could and did contrive Cromwell's decapitation. Henry lived with Anne of Cleves only a few months. She was so grateful to him for divorce instead of the executioner's block that she did everything within her power to expedite the disunion. Both Henry and Anne averred that her virginity had not been disturbed. The affair had many of the elements of comic opera.

On the day Cromwell was beheaded, Henry celebrated the event by taking his fifth bride, Catherine Howard, an animated little flapper with the glitter of a jewel and the morals of a female guttersnipe. Upon Henry she had the rejuvenating effect of a course of androgenic hormones until he learned that she was flirting openly with the young men of the court. She confessed illicit relations and was sent to the headsman forthwith.

It is an interesting fact that, though Henry was quite unmanageable during the decade of 1536–46, frequently spurning his constituted advisors and condemning his best friends, he never showed other traits suggestive of mental impairment. The age of fifty found him, except for his official rigidity, a mellow and, for his time, a benign and even generous monarch. Although Catherine

Howard had deceived him as no other woman ever had done, it was the councilors and not Henry who sent her to her death. After Catherine had been disposed of, the Parliament decreed it lawful for any person to inform on any lightness of the queen "for the time being." Also a screening statute was enacted declaring guilty of high treason any unchaste woman who should venture into marriage with the King. Henry, apparently, did not resent the implication of unfitness to manage his matrimonial affairs. Rather, he seemed to view the enactments as he would view guarantees of the worthiness of an article purchased in the market. Never before had he displayed such political astuteness. He proclaimed justice and no persecution for every subject in his realm; he won the loyalty of insurgent North England; he placated the Scotch; and he made English noblemen out of "Irish savages." He continued, however, to hate the Pope with an unremitting hatred, and he was waging an unpopular war against the French. In 1544 he was able to go before Parliament and defend his conduct of the war with such tender and ingratiating eloquence that at the end he had half the members crying like whipped children.

On July 12, 1543, Henry was married to Catherine Parr, who, offspring being out of the question, addressed her energy to the task of babying her husband and making him more comfortable. Catherine was a noblewoman twice a widow and of unassailable character.

By mid-year 1546 all was not well with Henry. He now had multiple leg ulcers which pained and stunk and had to be dressed several times daily. His growing irascibility was aggravated by political and religious contention. At one time he went so far as to denounce Catherine for attempting, by intercession, to temper justice with mercy and for differing with him on certain minor tenets of religion. In his rage he signed an indictment against her, but his heart had softened by the time the guard arrived to carry her away.

By November his dropsy was far advanced: his legs were elephantine, his body as big as that of a horse. He is said to have weighed more than four hundred pounds. At the new year, 1547, he could walk only a few steps; on the evening of January 27 it was apparent that dissolution was near. He was brought a death warrant to sign against the loyal old Norfolk who was in the Tower charged with conspiracy, but the great monarch could not lift a hand. Archbishop Cranmer, just arrived, rushed in to talk with him, but his Majesty was too drowsy. He must have a little sleep, then he would attend to Norfolk and the matter of his own immortal soul. His sleep deepened into coma, there was a brief struggle, and he breathed no more. Norfolk was relieved; the Archbishop, pensive.

Since the duration of his dropsy was only about six months and nothing is said to indicate that he suffered from the extreme orthopnea[1] so characteristic of heart failure, we infer that Henry had cirrhosis of the liver with obstruction of the portal system of veins, so-called hepatic dropsy. Whether his cirrhosis was of the alcoholic or syphilitic type is anybody's guess. He had earned the right to both types.

[1] Inability to breathe except in the upright position.

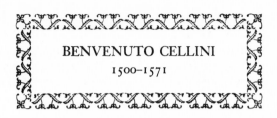

BENVENUTO CELLINI
1500–1571

H AD BENVENUTO CELLINI lived in any other age in history or in any other country than Italy, he could not possibly have been the man whom he portrays so divertingly in his *Autobiography*. It is doubtless true that genius carries its own inspiration, but it is also true that genius does not carry its own opportunities for expression. Perhaps the greatest ultimate value of the Cellini document lies in the remarkable clarity with which it illuminates a period unique in the history of the world.

It was in Italy and in Cellini's time that the smoldering fires of the Renaissance suddenly blazed forth in their fullest splendor. "The Italians," says Symonds, "were the first-born among the sons of modern Europe." The Italian, Christopher Columbus, had stirred the imaginations of men by flouting the ancient precepts of navigation to sail unimagined distances and discover strange lands and strange people; Copernicus was boldly mapping the sacred heavens; Leonardi da Vinci with the most versatile of minds was opening up new vistas in both art and science; and Vesalius, breaking with medical tradition, was exposing the errors of Galen while conducting his own revealing studies in human anatomy. At the same time, the physicians of Italy more than any others were rationalizing the practice of medicine.

It is noteworthy that Cellini in his many recorded episodes of illness never hesitated to call upon physicians for aid. True, he frequently disagreed with them, sometimes with a preponderance of reason on his side. But he rested his faith in *materia medica* and surgery and he wanted no mysticism or hocus pocus either for himself or for others. When his eyes became so inflamed that in his words, "I expected for certain to be left without my eyesight," he cured himself by bathing them with a decoction of fleur-de-lis, "stock, blossom, and root together." And writing of his brother Cecchino, who had suffered a gunshot wound of the lower thigh in an affray, Benvenuto remarks, "The doctors consulted together and treated him but they could not make up their minds to cut off his leg else perchance they might have saved him."

Whenever Cellini became acutely ill, he immediately despaired of recovery and in a state of utter despondency endeavored to reconcile himself to his expected fate. Once, after a night of pleasure, several boils appeared on his left forearm. The plague was rampant in the country at the time and Benvenuto concluded at once that he had fallen a victim to that dread disease. A physician was summoned who seemed to concur in the diagnosis, but was unable to reassure the patient with respect to the probable outcome. Shortly, however, "the admirable remedies which were applied" did their work and the terrified artist recovered from his furunculosis.

Of the greatest medical interest is Cellini's account of his syphilis. When he was about twenty-five years of age, he broke out with the "French disease," appropriately so called because it was brought to Italy and disseminated among the population by the soldiers of Charles VIII of France. Cellini wrote his own case history in these words: "It was true indeed that I had got the sickness, but I believe I caught it from that fine young servant-girl whom I was keeping when my house was robbed. The French disease, for it was that, remained in me four months dormant before it showed itself and then it broke out over my whole body at one instant. It was not like what one commonly observes but covered my flesh with certain blisters of the size of six-pences and rose colored.[1] The doctors would not call it the French disease,

---

[1] The Symonds translation is "blisters," but the MacDonell rendition is "red boils." The latter is probably nearer the true description since blisters would not likely have a rose color. Dark red papules are common in early cutaneous syphilis; real blisters occur almost exclusively in the congenital form of the disease.

albeit I told them why I thought it was that. I went on treating myself according to their methods but derived no benefit. At last, then, I resolved on taking the wood against the advice of the first physicians in Rome, and I took it with the most scrupulous discipline and rules of abstinence that could be thought of, and after a few days I perceived in me a great amendment. The result was that at the end of fifty days I was cured and as sound as a fish in water."

Just why Cellini believed the disease had lain dormant four months allows of two possible explanations: He may have been reckoning from what he considered the date of first exposure to the date of first appearance of the skin rash, but it seems more likely that he was counting from the time the presence of the initial sore (chancre) was first noted and that was the reason which he gave the doctors for thinking he had syphilis. All this happened about the year 1525 when physicians were just beginning to suspect the venereal origin of the disease. The significance of the chancre was then a matter of dispute and the great diversity of the skin manifestations was not yet appreciated. The disease could hardly have lain dormant more than three months after it was contracted, but four months would be about an average interval of time between the first appearance of the primary sore and the advent of the secondary skin rash.

When Cellini writes of "taking the wood," he is referring to guaiac wood, the heart wood of *Guaiacum officinale* or *G. sanctum*, certain flowering trees found in tropical America and the source of the drug Guaiac. Sollman's *Manual of Pharmacology* describes guaiac as "an almost obsolete remedy for syphilis, gout, rheumatism, tuberculosis, etc. . . . introduced soon after the discovery of America, about 1501–1503. Nicholaus Pohl (1517) stated that it had cured three thousand Spaniards. Its popularity was proclaimed in a famous pamphlet of Ulrich von Hutten, 1519. It was still strongly endorsed by Boerhaave (1668–1738) who wrote that 'it will act as a purge, reaching places that mercury cannot reach, and there dissolve the poison.' As early as 1538 Ruiz Diaz de Isla gave the credit to the associated regimen and indeed von Hutten had some suspicion in this direction."

The fact that to some Cellini's vainglory has seemed of

pathological proportions, coupled with a fairly definite history of syphilis, has caused speculation whether he may have had paretic dementia, a type of late syphilis of the brain frequently associated with an expansive egoism which manifests itself in delusions of grandeur and great self-esteem. In a personal conversation, the late Richard C. Cabot, professor of medicine at Harvard, expressed an emphatic opinion that Cellini did not have cerebral syphilis in any degree or form. Few of those whose clinical and literary experience qualifies them to speak on the subject will disagree with Dr. Cabot. They know too well that syphilis is a destroyer of genius and a mortal enemy of artistic and intellectual achievement.

There is no available evidence to indicate that Cellini had active syphilis beyond the first few months after the disease was contracted. His good fortune may be ascribed to two circumstances. First is the clinical observation that syphilis with early cutaneous manifestations has a notably lower incidence of late, so-called third-stage syphilis, especially of the nervous and cardiovascular systems. Whether this phenomenon is due to a less virulent strain of the infecting organism in the first place or to more effective antibody formation by the integument is not known. Second is the beneficent action of fever on the clinically syphilitic patient. Fever therapy, as everyone knows, is widely used in present-day treatment of late neurosyphilis and it is occasionally used to abort early syphilis. Cellini tells of a severe attack of fever of several days' duration which seized him not long after his skin rash had appeared. It followed exposure to wintry winds and water and probably was due to an acute infection in the upper respiratory tract, or what is now commonly called "flu."

At the age of thirty-five, Cellini was laid low by a fever of more than two months' duration. At one time he was thought to be dying, and some of his friends, eager to be the first to break the news, reported that he was dead. He tells of his persistent delirium and how he was endlessly harassed by hallucinations of an old man who wished to carry him off in a boat. It is probable that this illness was either typhoid or typhus fever; and if at its beginning there were any virulent treponemas in his system, they were, at the end, either destroyed by the inordinate temperature or rendered harmless by its attenuating action.

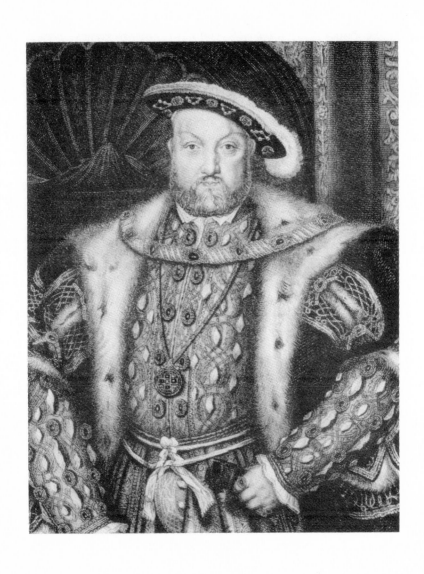

HENRY VIII

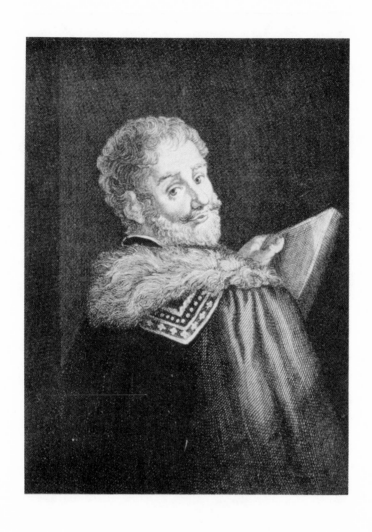

BENVENUTO CELLINI

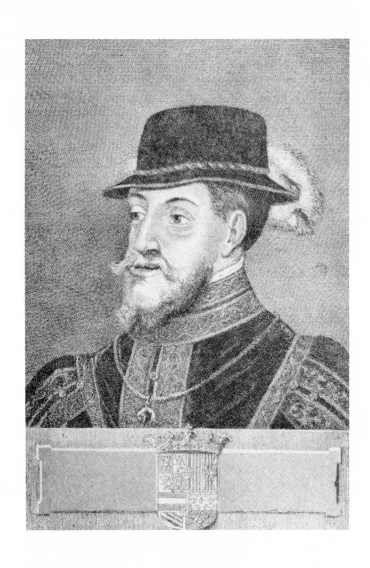

PHILIP II

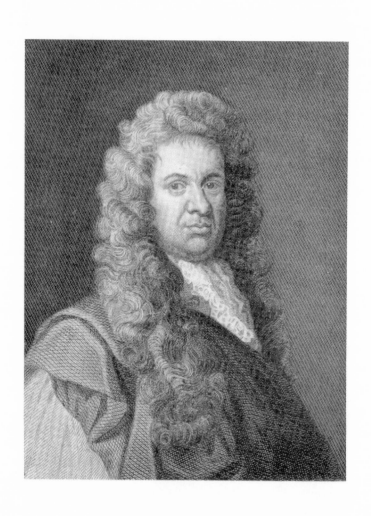

SAMUEL PEPYS

Cellini's panicky reaction to illness suggests that he was basically something of a coward. But he had what amounted to a faculty for rage which, in the presence of his enemies, enabled him to swallow his fear and perform deeds of considerable daring. His life was a succession of imbroglios and brawls. He boasted of three murders, one of which he says was unintentional. His morals were perhaps a little under the prevailing low level of his time. His Pharasaic declaration that men of genius are "above the law" was probably a sop to his own conscience quite as much as it was an appeal for the indulgent judgment of others, for he wished to think of himself not only as a man of surpassing genius but as a person of honor and integrity as well.

Readers of the *Autobiography* who are puzzled to know how much of it can be accepted as truth may find a modicum of reassurance in the fact that much of the material having to do with persons and places, comings and goings, events and occasions, has been checked and found to be surprisingly accurate. Some of his statements, particularly those involving his skill and prowess, are obvious falsifications. For example, he certainly pulls the long bow, perhaps we should say the long arquebus, when he tells of how with that primitive firearm he was able to perform feats of marksmanship which would be the envy of a modern expert rifleman using the best of present-day equipment. His tale of how he bethought himself to use "a noiseless kind of powder," impliedly of his own invention, for potshooting the Cardinal's peacocks is a poacher's dream and nothing more.

At the age of sixty-five, feeling the encroachments of age and the need for tender care, Cellini was married to Piera di Salvadore Parigi, who had once been his servant and mistress. Throughout his remaining years his artistic and social activities are said to have been sadly restricted by chronic arthritis. Early in the year 1571 he was stricken with "pleurisy." Since physicians of the time did not distinguish between uncomplicated pleurisy which rarely kills, and pleuro-pneumonia which kills very often, we may conjecture that it was the latter which on February 13 of the year indicated brought the calm of death to the tempestuous life of Benvenuto Cellini.

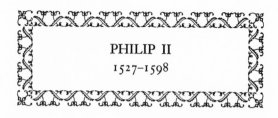

PHILIP II
1527–1598

WHEN the sick and frustrated Charles V. King of Spain and emperor of the Holy Roman Empire, abdicated his Spanish throne in favor of his son, Philip, he gilded the occasion with these words: "If the vast possessions which are now bestowed on you had come by inheritance, there would be much cause for gratitude. How much more when they come as a free gift in the lifetime of your father!" Presumably, Charles meant to congratulate Philip as a lucky fellow who was privileged both to have his paternal cake and to eat it.

As it turned out, the new king had very little cause for gratitude. But it was his manifest destiny to rule Spain, and, relying upon God's favor, he confidently assumed the burden cast off by the old monarch. To the difficult problems of sovereignty, the twenty-nine-year-old Philip brought the greatest piety, determination, and industry. Eventually, by the exercise of unparalleled religious and political despotism, he managed to add substantially to the legacy of trouble bequeathed him by his father.

Philip is best remembered for his zealous prosecution of the Inquisition in the Netherlands, his conflicts with the Popes, expulsion of the Moors and Jews from Spain, and the disastrous defeat suffered by the Invincible Armada which he launched against England. Historians are generally agreed that the decline of Spain as a great power had its beginning in the reign of Philip II.

38

It was six years after his accession that Philip felt the first twinges of an acute malady which was to become chronic a decade later and hound him to his grave. He steadfastly regarded his affliction as God's rebuke to a servant who was not properly diligent in the holy work of exterminating heretics and winning converts to the one true faith. His disease is, therefore, of historical importance because it largely explains the unspeakable cruelties inflicted by a man who was not basically inhumane upon the hapless victims of the Spanish Inquisition.

Philip's malady was gouty-arthritis, the same disease that killed his father two years after relinquishing his throne. Gout, in its commonest form, is not considered a fatal disorder. Once it has advanced to the stage of gouty-arthritis, however, with deposits of urates in and about the joints, the mortality rate, even today, is significant. The course of the disease is one of great chronicity marked by frequent relapses and remissions with hideous deformity and severe disability. Death may ensue from associated coronary or cerebro-vascular disease, kidney stone, intercurrent infections, bedsores, and general exhaustion. Ninety-five per cent of its victims are males and in half the cases there is a family history of the disease, often extending back several generations. Other factors than heredity which may play a role in the incidence and severity of the disease are diet, alcoholism, trauma, occupation, climate, race, and age. Remarkably enough, the early stages of the malady are much more painful than the later stages.

In person, Philip was of slight physique and serious mien. He is said to have been rigidly abstemious and "less immoral than most kings of his time." He possessed a tremendous capacity for work, but, strangely, his besetting fault as an administrator was procrastination. In Philip the deeply rooted philosophy of *mañana* flowered and bore its bitterest fruit. Frequently, after receiving a report demanding an immediate decision, he would fiddle away precious hours or days re-editing the manuscript or correcting the grammar of the writer while the couriers and generals waited impatiently for instructions. At St. Quentin, after Savoy had defeated and scattered the French army and Europe lay in the palm of Philip's hand, he could not make up his mind to grasp it. Anger, and anger alone, could galvanize him into prompt action.

39

As a youth Philip was well instructed in fencing, riding, and the "chivalrous exercises familiar to cavaliers of the time." Also "he was encouraged to invigorate his constitution with the hardy pleasures of the chase," but following his accession he seems to have renounced such physical frivolities for the minutiae of absolute dictatorship.

For the next thirty-five years following his initial attack of gout, Philip's medical history revolves about that ailment. Almost imperceptibly the attacks increased in frequency and severity, but no serious disability was manifest until he was about sixty-five years of age. Meantime he had a few attacks of malaria, although in general he seems to have been remarkably free of infectious disorders.

It has frequently been stated in the delicate phraseology of writers who flourished before our present age of medical frankness that Philip suffered from the "sins of his father" or that he had a "loathsome hereditary disease," meaning, no doubt, syphilis. There is also a tendency among modern writers to explain every affliction or premature death among royalty of the period by the generalization that "they were all syphilitic." All experienced physicians know that mass diagnosis is dangerous and that each case must be considered in the light of the patient's symptoms. In the case of Philip, in contrast to that of Henry VIII, for example, there is no convincing evidence of syphilis in either his personal history or his marital record.

Philip had four wives in all, each of whom passed on before her master. His first wife was María, a Portuguese princess who died eleven months after their marriage and three days after presenting her husband with a male heir. According to the chroniclers of the time her death resulted from "imprudently eating a lemon." The second wife was Mary Tudor, congenitally syphilitic daughter of Henry VIII of England and Catherine of Aragon. Bloody Mary, who apparently was sterile, died of apoplexy at the age of forty-two. The third wife was Elizabeth de Valois, who yielded two living daughters and a few days before her queenly demise from a fever (probably either typhus or typhoid) suffered miscarriage of a third girl. The fourth and last of Philip's wives was Anne of Austria, a marvel of fertility who in a decade gave birth to six living children and lost another by miscarriage. Of the six, only one attained maturity—a commentary on the child mortality rate of the time.

Don Carlos, Philip's son by his first wife, María, has been the subject of much speculative writing. There can be no doubt that he was physically and mentally abnormal, but there is no good evidence that he was born syphilitic. He has been described as lame, stunted, epileptic, spindly legged, and possessed of an abnormally large head. The last two attributes are suggestive of hydrocephalus. He is said to have fallen from a ladder in his teens and hurt his head, following which injury erysipelas supervened. The sick prince was delirious for weeks. An Italian surgeon was called in who diagnosed a brain injury and performed a trephine of the skull without immediate success. Finally the priests took over and had the bones of Fray Diego, a holy man who had died a hundred years before, dug up and placed in bed with the sick prince. Improvement followed promptly, affording, perhaps, the earliest recorded evidence of the value of shock-therapy. A heated argument ensued between the physicians and the clergy, with each group claiming credit for the cure. The dispute was gently resolved when Carlos suddenly evinced a homicidal mania which made it necessary to place him in confinement. He died in prison at the age of twenty-three under circumstances which have never been fully revealed.

In his late sixties, Philip's illness was plainly entering its final stage. One arm was practically useless, a knee was bent and rigid, and he was able to hobble about the palace only with the greatest difficulty. Although he certainly suffered some pain and a great deal of inconvenience, he was never heard to utter a word of complaint. At the age of seventy, he was practically bedfast. He was barely able to feed himself and was quite unable to dress or to care for his toilet. The surgeons bled him unmercifully and also treated the swollen knee locally, probably by the insertion of setons which produced numerous open sores about the joint. As a result of this infection the king's naturally meager body was further shrunken by toxemia and fever.

Philip desired to celebrate his seventy-first birthday with a grand ball. Since he could not attend a ball, he had the ball attend him; it was held in the royal apartment where, with his head propped up on a pillow against which he looked like a gnome, the sick little man watched the ladies and gentlemen move through the graceful measures of the dances. A few weeks later he desired to be moved to the huge Escorial, the combined palace, church, school, and monastery which he had built to honor God for the victory He had given Spanish arms at St. Quentin. In order to avoid painful jolting as far as possible, Philip was carried the entire twenty-seven miles by relays of litter-bearers. There he was placed on a couch so situated that he could look into the church and view the altar. Throughout the final two months of his illness he lay thus, murmuring prayers or listening to the monks as they chanted hymns which were pleasing to God.

To the infected sores made by the setons were added bedsores and sundry ulcerations so that he could be neither moved nor bathed because of the pain caused by such procedures. At any rate he was spared one annoyance; the appalling stench repelled all curious visitors. On the evening of September 12, 1598, it was noted that he seemed weaker than usual, and by midnight it was apparent that the end was only a few hours away. The patient himself must have realized it, too, for just before the rising sun began to streak the sky, he asked for the little wooden crucifix which his father, Emperor Charles, had held in his last moment of life. At the instant of sunrise, with the tiny emblem of his faith tightly clutched in his bloodless fingers, Philip II, king of Spain, expired.

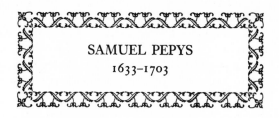

I<small>N MATTERS</small> of the health and medical interests of its author, the diary of the Honorable Samuel Pepys partakes of the peculiarities which characterize the journal as a whole. The amusing small talk, the confessions, and the self-reproach without true penitence when indulgence brought physical pain, are all in character with the man we know as Pepys.

The diary compasses a single period of exactly ten years and five months, beginning a few weeks before Pepys' twenty-seventh birthday. Since he died at the age of seventy, it is obvious that for material relating to the six other decades of his life, his biographers must look elsewhere than to the diary. Moreover, the diary is not completely informative even for its own time.

Pepys' declared reason for terminating the diary was his failing eyesight. He abandoned the work in the belief that he was faced by complete loss of vision. The final entry concludes with the sentence, "And so I betake myself to that course which is almost as much as to see myself go into my grave, for which and all the discomforts that will accompany my being blind, the good God prepare me!" Happily, the gloomy prophecy failed of fulfillment and if, eventually, he ceased to appreciate a well-turned ankle or a comely feminine figure, the fault was not in the organs of sight.

There is abundant evidence that Pepys' visual troubles were due to astigmatism coupled with eyestrain. He used small tube-

spectacles for reading and found them helpful because they eliminated some of the scattered rays which his astigmatic eyes were
unable to converge to a focal point. His constant reading and writing under conditions of poor illumination imposed a strain with
which his congenitally defective eyes could not cope. The left
eye—as often happens in the case of a right-handed person—was
weaker than the right and consequently, was "more watery."
Eventually, he appealed to his friend, Cocker, a genius of sorts,
who fitted him with green spectacles which are said to have lessened the painful effects of light and to have sharpened his vision a
little. He was probably about forty years of age at this time, and
hyperopia, a condition of reduced perception for near objects and
commonly known as "far-sightedness," could have added to his
distress. The green glasses may have carried some degree of correction for far-sightedness since spectacles for the relief of that
condition were commonly used long before the time of Pepys. It
was not until 1825, however, that the nature of astigmatism was
first revealed, by Sir George B. Airy, and it was more than a half-
century later before glasses for correction of the condition were
commonly prescribed.

For most of his life Pepys suffered from urinary calculi—
kidney and bladder stones. This affliction was the curse of his existence. It compelled him, in desperation, to submit to the very
formidable operation of being "cut for the stone" at the age of
twenty-two, and it finally caused his death after fifty years of
intermittent suffering and ill health. Strangely, the disorder seems
to have run in the family. Pepys states that when he visited his
mother in 1660, she was "in greater and greater pain of the stone."
He tells also of his aunt at Brompton who "voided a great stone"
and of his brother, John, who had just donned his bachelor's cap
at Cambridge and who "hath the stone and makes bloody water
with great pain."

The identity of the surgeon who operated upon Pepys is not
positively known, but he is believed to have been Thomas Hollis-
ter, lithotomist at St. Bartholomew's Hospital at the time. The
operation was done at the house of a Mrs. Turner, and the site of
the scar, as revealed at necropsy, indicated that the surgeon had
used the lateral-perineal approach to the bladder, a technique de-

vised by the great French surgeon, Ambrose Pare. John Evelyn, probably Pepys' closest friend, relates that the stone was the size of a tennis ball, which would indicate a weight of about two ounces. For many years Pepys celebrated the twenty-sixth of March as a feast day "for my being cut of the stone." The operation unquestionably gave him great relief, though he continued to pass an occasional gravel and suffered repeated attacks of a colic which he did not recognize as due to stone in a kidney. He did note, however, that after a convivial evening he was likely to have pain in the groin and burning on urination the following day, and he wished that he had the good sense to practice abstinence.

For a time he took daily doses of turpentine to forestall attacks of colic. As turpentine is notoriously irritating to the kidneys, it would seem that his choice of a remedy was not a happy one. He also carried a rabbit's foot and, having suffered attacks of colic despite the charm, was about to lose faith in it when a Mr. Batten showed him that "the hare's foot hath not a joint in it" and consequently should not be expected to perform effectively. He immediately procured another which conformed to the Batten specifications.

Shortly before Pepys began his diary, he "had a boil under the chin which troubled me cruelly." As the boil failed to heal satisfactorily, he came to the alarming conclusion that he had cancer. He was reassured by a visit to Mr. Fage, the surgeon, who gave him "something for it."

Pepys' wife died of a fever, believed to have been typhoid, in 1669 at the age of twenty-nine years. In their nearly fifteen years of married life, she was never pregnant. D'Arcy Power, eminent British surgeon, believed that the operation which Pepys underwent for removal of the bladder stone had rendered him sterile. He was never married again.

In his post-diary years Pepys had minor ailments unrelated to his kidney and bladder troubles. He suffered frequent attacks of indigestion caused by surfeits of rich food. Once after a visit to Epsom and a round of purging, he developed a strangulated hemorrhoid which he greatly feared might prove to be a rupture—an absurd notion, of course, arising from his total lack of surgical knowledge. He was continually catching colds which he ascribed to exposure of his head incidental to a fresh haircut, leaving off his periwig, or sitting at dinner without his hat. His excessive sensitivity in this respect suggests the presence of a chronic sinus infection. He also had attacks of "nettle-rash" each fall coincident with the onset of cold weather. A likely explanation is that he was allergic to his "woolens."

Pepys' insatiable curiosity led to an interest in animal experimentation. He describes a "pretty experiment" at Gresham College in November, 1666, in which "the blood of one dog let out till he died, into the body of another on one side while all his own ran out on the other side. The first died upon the place and the other very well and likely to do well." He tells also of going with Dr. Pierce "to see an experiment of killing a dog by letting opium into his hind leg." He and Dr. Clerk "did fail mightily of hitting the vein but with the little they got in did presently fall asleep." In a third experiment which he describes but apparently did not see, sheep's blood was said to have been transfused into the veins of a debauched fellow with resultant amelioration of the recipient's character. The fact that the man survived indicates that very little if any of the sheep's blood entered his circulatory system, though the experience may have sufficed to teach him a lesson.

Pepys' death evidently resulted from his urinary tract disorder. It may have been due to uremia, the result of suppressed kidney function. A necropsy was done, the exact findings of which are not recorded. It is said that there were evidences of senile arteriosclerosis, which was to be expected, and for a certainty a number of stones were found in the left kidney. Undoubtedly the stone which was removed by operation at Mrs. Turner's had its beginning as a kidney gravel which descended into the bladder and there grew to its great size by the accretion of urinary salts. Had Pepys lived in our time, his trouble could have been completely eradicated by surgery and his life made much more comfortable thereby. It is greatly to his credit that, feeling the approach of death, he readily gave his consent for a post-mortem dissection of his body.

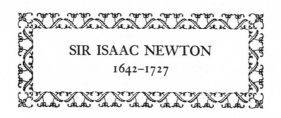

Mathematics is a high-level system of thinking, and the true mathematician is endowed with a special type of mind which reveals itself early in life. It was through no fault of Isaac Newton that the mathematical quality of his intellect went unrecognized until he reached the age of sixteen and had been kept out of school for a year. When a visiting uncle snatched a book from the boy's hand and found it to be a treatise on mathematics for university students, it must have been evident to him that Isaac had been thinking mathematically for some time. Otherwise he would not have interceded with the lad's mother to have her son returned to school.

Newton was born at Woolsthorpe, in the County of Lincoln, on Christmas Day, 1642. He is thought to have come into the world two or three weeks before he was due. If this belief is correct, it may account for his delicate babyhood and early childhood. His father had died several months before Isaac was born, and when, after three years of widowhood, the mother was married to a local rector, the care of the child passed into the hands of his grandmother who lived near by. Eventually the boy was sent to local schools for instruction and, at the age of twelve, to the town of Grantham for further education. Through the first year at Grantham he was regarded as one of the poorest students in his class, and in the second year he did no better, so the story goes, until the school bully dealt him a heavy blow in the stomach. Then, aroused but despairing of his ability to take revenge in kind, young Newton decided to humiliate the fellow by outstripping him in his studies. To the discomfiture of the enemy and the astonishment of the teacher, Isaac became the school's outstanding pupil.

Our credulity is further taxed by the tale of how, a dozen years later, a falling apple banged the Newtonian head and set it pondering the mysteries of gravitation. It is apparent that, as a result of the two miraculous blows suffered by Isaac, the hard shell which imprisoned his genius was cracked wide open.

After he had completed three years at Grantham, the lad's schooling was interrupted at the command of his mother, who, having lost her second husband, felt that her son's help was required at home on the farm. It is said that he was a good boy, but his preoccupation with mechanical toys and "cyphers" caused his mother a certain amount of vexation. Apparently, however, she had no intention of sending Isaac back to school until her brother persuaded her to do so. The lad returned to Grantham, where he remained until he reached the age of eighteen and had qualified for admission to Trinity College at Cambridge.

The eminent Dr. Barrow was professor of mathematics in Trinity College at that time, and to prepare himself for Barrow's lectures, Newton set to work on Saunderson's *Logic*, Kepler's *Treatise on Optics*, Descartes' *Geometry*, and Wallis' *De Arithmetica Infinitorum*. He mastered those works quickly and was welcomed to Barrow's classes, where, under the guidance of the great teacher, he began his historic explorations into the hinterland of mathematics.

In January, 1665, Newton received the degree of Bachelor of Arts and then promptly fled Cambridge to escape the great epidemic of bubonic plague which was devastating South England at the time. This was the epidemic which is described in lurid detail by Daniel Defoe in his *Journal of the Plague Year* and by Samuel Pepys in his celebrated diary. During this absence, which covered a period of one and one-half years, Newton lived in laborious seclusion. When he emerged and returned to Cambridge, he brought with him two completely new methods of mathematical analysis, namely, differential and integral calculus and the famous Newtonian formula containing the essence of the Universal Law of Gravitation. Thus before his twenty-fourth birthday he had achieved a renown surpassing that of any other scientist of his time. The formula, however, added no part to the general acclaim as yet, since it was to undergo an extended period of probation before release.

At Cambridge he resumed his academic work and in 1669 succeeded to the professorship of mathematics and physics—the post being voluntarily vacated by Dr. Barrow, who wished to devote himself to theology. Newton's health must have remained quite good, for in the next twenty-three years no mention is made of illness, and, moreover, except for the regular annual vacation, the record shows no absence from the university during the period. The faculty of Cambridge was permitted a representative in Parliament, and in 1688 Newton was chosen for the honor, which he retained until 1695, the maximum life of a parliament being seven years at that time instead of the present five years.

At first he was disposed to take his official duties seriously and rarely missed a sitting. Later, however, his interest languished, and the final three years of his term were marked by frequent absences. In the latter part of the year 1692 a disastrous fire in his home destroyed records containing all the accumulated data of several years' experimental work in chemistry. To this shocking misfortune is ascribed a mental illness which appeared not long after and persisted for eighteen months. The biographer Biot states that Newton was actually insane during most of 1693–94. Biot's allegation is vigorously assailed by Sir David Brewster, who wrote the standard biography of the great mathematician. In defense of Newton's sanity Sir David submits two letters written by Newton during the period of his disquietude. They were addressed to John Locke (who had just published a second edition of his *On Human Understanding*) and, it would seem, do Sir David's argument no good whatever. The first of the letters follows:

> Sir: Being of opinion that you endeavored to embroil me with women and by other means, I was so much affected with it as that when one told me you were sickly and would not live, I answered, "twere better you were dead." I desire you to forgive me this uncharitableness, for I am now satisfied

that what you have done is just, and I beg your pardon for having bad thoughts of you for it and for representing that you struck at the roots of morality in principle you laid in your book of ideas and designed to pursue in another book and that I took you for a Hobbist. I beg your pardon also, for saying or thinking there was a desire to sell me an office or to enbroil me.

I am your most humble and unfortunate servant, Is. Newton.

It is by no means unusual for the author of a new book to receive a complaint from some obscure lunatic who imagines himself the object of laborious defamation, but Locke must have been amazed at a letter of that sort from Newton. On October 5, Locke replied, assuring Newton of his friendship and offering to go to him, "for the conclusion of your letter makes me apprehend that it would not be wholly valueless to you." Locke was a physician as well as a writer on philosophy, and seeing the evidence of despair and aberration in his friend, he desired to help him. Newton replied at once, saying:

Sir: The last winter by sleeping too often by my fire I got an ill habit of sleeping, and a distemper which this summer has been epidemical put me farther out of order so that when I wrote you I had not slept an hour a night for a fortnight together, and for five days together not a wink. I remember that I wrote to you but what I said of your book, I remember not. If you please to send me a transcript of that passage I will give you an account of it if I can. I am your most humble servant, Is. Newton.

The first letter bears the imprint of a persecution complex which, however, may have had a remote relationship to fact.

Newton had a niece who was a young woman of great beauty and charm. The two were very fond of each other, and it is said that certain jealous persons circulated a report that he had used his niece's favors to gain advantages which he could not have won on his merits. When news of this slander came to Sir Isaac's ears, as it had done some months previously, he was greatly perturbed. The allusion to a desire to sell him an office and to embroil him with women is merely a bit of memorial debris whirling about in the stream of confused consciousness. Locke always held Newton in the highest esteem, and since there was no conflict of interest between them, there was no reason for jealousy. Moreover, Newton, by his own words, was physically sick. What the "distemper" was which was "epidemical" that summer is not clear, but it was probably either an intestinal or a respiratory infection. It seems evident that he suffered from a psychosis due to infectious disease with possible vitamin deficiency superimposed on nervous fatigue due to worry.

Whether Newton was or was not technically insane for a time is unimportant. Insanity is a legal and social rather than a medical term and implies mental lapse from a state of ability to manage one's affairs and to perform one's social duties. His disorder was not purely psychogenic since it was not cyclic or deteriorative; there was no return of the trouble and his old age was marked by extraordinary mental vigor. It is said that Liebnitz contrived a problem as a challenge to the mathematicians of Europe. Newton was apprised of the nature of the problem about five o'clock one evening after he had come home fatigued with a day's work in a public office. Next morning he mailed the correct solution to Liebnitz with thanks for a good night's sleep. At that time Newton was seventy-four years of age.

It is regrettable that Newton was not provided with a subsidy to enable him to pursue his scientific studies. The fact that he had to pay for experimental equipment out of his own pocket, which he could not afford, was probably the sole reason for his apparent loss of zest for research while he was still in the prime of intellectual life. As a member of Parliament and warden of the Mint he became a victim of what Bell terms "the crowning imbecility of the Anglo-Saxon breed," which he defines as "its dumb belief in public office or an administrative function as the supreme honor for a man of intellect."

In 1699, Sir Isaac was made director of the Mint with the comfortable salary of £1,500 annually. Unfortunately, the demands of the directorship were so great that he felt obligated to resign his professorship in order to care for the "King's business." In 1701 he was again elected to Parliament and in 1703 he was made president of the Royal Society of London, a position which he held the remainder of his life.

In person, Newton was medium in height and, in his later years, inclined to stoutness. Bishop Atterbury asserts that during the last twenty years of life the great mathematician's eyes had a dull, tired expression. During his years of research he was extremely absent-minded and would sometimes sit on the side of his bed half-dressed for hours at a time. When, however, he became director of the Mint, he lost his preoccupation with science and became an alert and practical-minded administrator. There is evidence that Flamsteed, director of the Greenwich Observatory, spoke with some justice when he described Newton as "invidious, ambitious, exceedingly avid of praise, and very irritable when contradicted." He was thrifty and became moderately wealthy in late middle age. He was a lifelong bachelor, he never wore glasses, and his teeth were sound and serviceable to the day of his death.

Sir Isaac is said to have enjoyed fair health and never to have been seriously ill until the age of eighty-three. Then he began to suffer acute attacks of pain, the location of which is not indicated. The paroxysms increased in severity until, in the last months of his life, he would sit pale and impassive, his face covered with cold sweat. The doctors diagnosed his trouble as "the stone." Since there is no mention of urinary disturbance, the physicians probably had kidney or ureteral stone in mind. It appears that the diagnosis was based entirely on the apparent severity of the pain. Fontenelle is quoted as saying in his *Éloge de Newton*, "Twas thought he certainly had the stone which could not be cured, when the pain was so violent that drops of sweat ran from his face." About three weeks before his death the pain left him and he expired peacefully on March 20, 1727, at the age of eighty-four.

The probable cause of his pain was angina pectoris, symptomatic of the coronary artery disease which was to cause his death. "Kidney colic" causes the patient to writhe and cry out in agony; severe angina transfixes its victim with pain and a sense of imminent dissolution. It often happens that the angina subsides a few days or weeks before the occurrence of exodus in fatal coronary disease. Moreover, even in Newton's day, when kidney stone was much more common in England than now, there must have been many cases of coronary disease for every case of the stone.

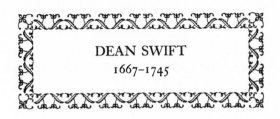

WITH THE SOLITARY EXCEPTION of Daniel De-
foe, no other eminent British author has written as voluminously
as Dean Swift. Perhaps none has written more brilliantly. But
Swift was a satirist, and fundamentally a satirist has two loves:
himself and his invidious art. The reading public has sensed this
truth and therein lies the chief reason why, that of all Swift's works,
only two, *Gulliver's Travels* and *A Modest Proposal,* are commonly known today.

The posthumous son of Jonathan Swift by Abigail Leicester,
Dean (Jonathan) Swift was born in Dublin, Ireland. After his
graduation from Trinity College he obtained his Master of Arts
degree at Oxford in 1692. Two years later he returned to Ireland,
and one year after that, having been ordained, he settled at Kilroot.
In 1701 he was awarded the degree of Doctor of Divinity by Dublin, and in 1713 he succeeded to the deanship of St. Patrick's.

It is well known that the cantankerous Dean, like Martin
Luther, suffered throughout his adult life from frequent attacks
of dizziness associated with disturbances of hearing. His biographers have assigned his troublesome symptoms to a variety of
causes, mostly, since he was a satirist and a cleric, of a defamatory
character such as gluttony, alcoholism, excessive venery, and syphilis. Medical opinion has been a little kinder in suspecting epileptic
vertigo, otosclerosis, and insanity. Swift's own writings record
attacks of gout, shingles, and colds, but his principal complaints

53

concern his giddiness and deafness. His explanation of the origin of his ailments, as embodied in a letter to a Mrs. Howard, is both ludicrous and pathetic. Referring back to the time when he was about twenty-three years of age, he says, "About two hours before you were born I got my giddiness by eating a hundred golden pippins at a time and when you were five-years-and-a-quarter old, bating two days, having made a fine seat about twenty miles farther in Surry where I used to read—and there I got my deafness and these two friends have visited me, one or other, every year since, and being old acquaintances, have now thought fit to come together."

On September 1, 1714, he wrote, "My head is pretty well, only a sudden turn at any time makes me feel giddy for a moment and sometimes it feels very stuffed but if it grows no worse I can bear it very well." Alas, it did grow worse, and the frequency and volume of the Dean's complaints grew with it over the next score of years. In 1720 he asked significantly, "What if I should add that once in five or six weeks I am deaf for three or four days?"

In 1727 he had an attack which he alleged was brought on by "cider, fruit, and champagne." Later he wrote, "I walk like a drunken man and am deafer than ever you knew me." And in 1733, "I am just recovering [from] two cruel indispositions of giddiness and deafness after seven months. I have got my hearing but the other still hangs about me and, I doubt, will ever leave me till I leave it."

In 1736 he suffered another extremely severe attack of dizziness and deafness. Writing to Pope, he declared that he was unable even to make conversation. It was in November of that same year, however, that he launched a powerful diatribe entitled *The Legion Club* against the Irish House of Commons in College Green. It was his last literary effort. In a letter to Sheridan in 1737, Swift recalled how in England while he was yet a lad in his teens, "I got a cold which gave me a deafness I could never clear myself of." His deafness was of the low-tone type as evidenced by his statement, "I can hear with neither ear except it be a woman with a treble or a man with a counter tenor."

Dr. T. G. Wilson of Dublin, Ireland, in a discussion of Swift's deafness and giddiness makes a convincing diagnosis of the nature of the Dean's life-long ailment. Wilson rules out epilepsy, otosclerosis (bony ankylosis of the sound-conducting apparatus of the middle ear), and syphilitic labyrinthitis and clearly reveals that the Dean's unpleasant symptoms were due to an affection of the internal ear involving the organs of equilibrium and the auditory apparatus. This disorder, which is known as Ménière's disease, may be either chronic or recurrent. Some authorities hold that only the recurrent type should be called Ménière's disease. In the case of Swift, Dr. Wilson believed that a badly deflected nasal septum, revealed when the Dean's skull was disinterred nearly four-score years ago was, primarily, the source of his affliction. But modern medical teaching does not hold with the Doctor. Since the dizziness and the deafness seem to have come together and left together, Swift's case belongs in a category rather recently described by Drs. Sheldon and Horton of the Mayo Clinic. These workers have established that recurrent episodes of acute vertigo, ringing in the ear, and sudden deafness are commonly due to histamine sensitization (allergy) and are amenable to treatment designed to produce and maintain desensitization against the offending substance, whatever that substance may happen to be. If the Dean were living today, he could almost certainly obtain a high degree of relief from his giddiness and also, taken in time, his hearing might be preserved.

Vascular degenerative disease is one of the numerous attorneys of Nature whose function it is to foreclose the mortgage their client holds on every human life.

It was probably in the year 1736 that Swift first realized that he was being attacked by a new enemy when he noted a dulling of his memory and a slowing of his intellectual processes. He did not know, of course, that his attacker was cerebral arteriosclerosis of a special type with a hereditary propensity. In 1739 he wrote a lengthy composition of gloomy doggerel on the "Death of Doctor Swift," relating what he imagined his "special friends," as he termed them, were thinking and saying about him. Here he displays an acute awareness of his failing faculties and the inevitable issue of the infirmity, and he indicates that his greatest dread was not of death itself but rather of the satisfaction it might give his "special friends."

55

> *Though it is hardly understood*
> *Which way my death can do them good,*
> *Yet, thus methinks, I hear them speak:*
> *"See how the Dean begins to break*
> *Poor gentleman, he droops apace,*
> *You plainly see it in his face.*
> *That old vertigo in his head*
> *Will never leave him till he's dead.*
> *Besides, his memory decays,*
> *He recollects not what he says;*
> *He cannot call his friends to mind,*
> *Forgets the place where last he dined;*
> *Plyes you with stories o'er and o'er,*
> *He told them fifty times before.*
> *How does he fancy we can sit,*
> *To hear his out of fashioned wit?*
> *For poetry he's past his prime,*
> *He takes an hour to find a rime;*
> *His fire is out, his wit decay'd*
> *His fancy sunk, his muse a Jade.*
> *I'd have him throw away his pen,*
> *But there's no talking to some men."*

Swift furiously resisted the summons. He exercised to the limit of his endurance and he railed against his inability to recall names, dates, events, and finally the faces of long-time acquaintances. By 1742 he exhibited the typical symptoms of far-advanced cerebral arterial disease. "His comprehension and memory had failed so completely," says Wilson, "that he was incapable of conversation." In March of that year the Court of Chancery appointed guardians for the hapless Dean; five months later a commission declared him "of unsound mind and memory." On October 17, 1745, he was seized with convulsive fits which persisted for thirty-six hours. Then, after a few hours of quiet, he died.

A post-mortem examination was made by Mr. Whiteway, surgeon to St. Steeven's, but we learn only that the skull was opened and "there was much water in the brain." A death mask was made and, according to Sir Walter Scott, "the expression was unequivocally maniacal." Scott's statement is slightly ridiculous. Photographs of the mask accompanying Wilson's article suggest a slight degree of paralysis of the left side of the face, but otherwise, the expression is not unusual. Moreover, cerebral arteriosclerotics are not maniacal; they are confused and stuporous.

Had sections of the brain been made, they would probably have revealed extensive areas of subcortical softening with possible small hemorrhages and cyst formation. Since in this disease the arteries of the kidneys often show changes similar to those found in the brain, many cerebral arteriosclerotics die of uremic poisoning. The prolonged series of convulsive seizures just preceding death and the "wet brain" found post mortem suggest that Swift's death may have been of that order. More likely, however, the "much water" found by the autopsy surgeon was *around* the brain and not *in* the brain. In severe cases of cerebral arteriosclerosis a marked degree of atrophy of the brain is uniform in occurrence and the space vacated by the shrunken cerebrum is filled by a corresponding increase in the amount of cerebrospinal fluid.

There is, perhaps, an odd relevancy in the circumstance that in 1740, "being at this present of sound mind, although weak in body," the Dean executed his will by the terms of which his fortune, amounting to about eleven thousand pounds, was left to build a hospital for idiots and lunatics in the city of Dublin.

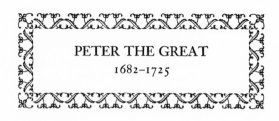

PETER THE GREAT
1682–1725

JOHN CHURCHILL, DUKE OF MARLBOROUGH, had occasion to visit Zaardam, Holland, in the year 1697. While inspecting the shipyards in that city, his attention was arrested by a workman of unusual appearance and manner. The fellow had an adze in his hand, and he wore a red woolen shirt, duck trousers, and a sailor's hat. He was powerfully built and his features were bold and regular. His hair was dark brown, his complexion ruddy, the veins of his neck distended, and his eyes were dark, keen, and restless. His voice was guttural but not unmusical. He seemed easily excited, tossed his arms about in violent gesticulation as he talked, and looked constantly as if he were about to give way to an explosion of passion or fall into a fit. Since his fellow workers appeared not to notice the man's apparent agitation, the Duke concluded that it was but the habitual expression of an intense and earnest nature. When the foreman commanded, "Carpenter Peter, help these men carry those planks," the nobleman, who had some pre-knowledge, concluded correctly that the person addressed was the Czar of Russia, Peter Alexievitch. A fellow workman of Peter's, a Dutch shipbuilder, gave a terse and significant description of the Czar when he wrote: "He is tall, with a head that shakes and a right arm that is never quiet. He has a wart on his right cheek." Czar Peter, who was twenty-four years of age at this time, had stopped at Zaardam in the course of an educational tour to gain firsthand experience in the art of constructing seaworthy ships—a task which he would thoroughly enjoy.

This extraordinary individual, who was born in or near Moscow, was the third son of Alexis Mihialovitch and the first child by his second wife, Natalia. Alexis died when Peter was but four years of age and the crown passed to Feodor, eldest son of Alexis and half-brother of Peter. Feodor was feeble in mind and body. Since he left no heir to succeed him on the throne, his death in 1682 fanned a smoldering family quarrel into a flaming revolution.

Ivan, the second son of Alexis, was sixteen years old at the time of Feodor's death and in the natural order of succession had first claim on the throne. However, he was a little too young, and what was much more serious, he was mentally deficient and subject to frequent seizures of epilepsy. Natalia wished to have Peter made czar to succeed Feodor, but was opposed by her stepdaughter, Sophia, third daughter of Alexis and hence half-sister of young Peter. Sophia rallied the Streltzy, or militia, to her cause and contrived to have Ivan proclaimed czar jointly with Peter, and herself elected regent. In effecting this coup, the Streltzy got completely out of hand, invaded the palace, seized Matveief, friend and counselor of Natalia, and hacked him to pieces before the horrified eyes of the ten-year-old Peter. Murder and pillage were rampant. At one time Peter was threatened but was spared, apparently because of his mother's pleadings. The bloody scenes which the boy witnessed and the terrors which he suffered that frightful night probably were an aggravating factor in certain nervous symptoms which appeared shortly and were to afflict him throughout the remainder of his life.

Peter's schooling was begun in his sixth year, but it was irregular, fragmentary, and ineffective. At the age of eleven, he had not yet learned to read or write. It is said that his tutor, Zutov, tried to instruct him in the history of Muscovy, but the lad was fidgety and inattentive. When however, a manuscript from the palace library was brought with pictures of the battlefields, the troops of both sides, and the generals, Peter was fascinated. He neither missed nor forgot any detail. His restless and wholly objective mind, oppressed by the restraints of the nursery and school, now found glorious release in the contemplation of action and

59

excitement of battle. His education had at last found its incentive. His memory of the Streltzy revolt was simply one of devils who came out of the dark to hack and tear hapless humans to bits. Now he saw war as a contest and armies as great machines by which highly desirable objectives might be attained. He wanted to play at war; to sniff the aroma but not yet to taste the substance.

Soon Peter, who was astonishingly large and strong for his years, was going on route marches in the country, sleeping on the ground, and living in genuine soldier fashion with his *"poteshny."* The latter constituted a sort of home guard which he had recruited from the idle grooms and falconers left lolling in obscene indolence around the stables of the deceased emperor, Alexis. They were companionable fellows who liked drinking and horseplay quite as much as they liked drilling and marching. Peter was well content to leave matters of state to sister Sophia. He desired only to play at soldiering. He and his *poteshny* accompanied the Streltzy on their marches, and the young militarist learned how to mend harness and to fix weapons in the army workshop. Eventually he had his own forge and shop and a marvelous machine of foreign make—a lathe. So zestful was life that the days were not half long enough. Only when he was penned up for a reading lesson or had to go to Moscow for a state function was he bored or unhappy. True, the nights were bad until he could go to sleep. When he was in camp with his *poteshny*, he was less afraid, but at home a peculiar terror would come out of the darkness. He could not sleep alone, so every night some luckless servant was chosen to occupy the bed with him. Peter usually slept with his head covered and pressed against the naked belly of his bedfellow. If the man dared move, the young Czar pummeled him with his fists. Occasionally Peter was laid up with what were called "spasms of the brain." Sometimes the attacks lasted only a few minutes, while at other times they were prolonged into hours or even days. His fifteenth year was marred by two violent seizures, each of which confined him to his room for several weeks. Throughout his life he was to suffer attacks of the malady in varying degrees of severity.

Peter had multiple disorders of the nervous system. He suffered from a fear complex, a hysteria possibly engendered by his shocking experiences during the revolt of the Streltzy in 1682, and from the age of fourteen he was a victim of habitual alcoholism and a peculiar type of epilepsy. To what extent his epileptic seizures were modified or aggravated by hysteria and alcoholism it is impossible to say. It is well known that hysteria may, on occasion, strongly simulate epilepsy, and it is also established that alcoholism may cause epileptiform seizures in persons not otherwise subject to them. Moreover, descriptions of Peter's attacks are so meager of detail that certain valuable diagnostic signs, if observed at all, were not recorded.

His half-brother Ivan was clearly epileptic and the other half-brother, Feodor, was little better than a high-grade imbecile. Epilepsy and feeble-mindedness tend to merge into a single hereditary trait. We may suppose, therefore, that since Peter, Ivan, and Feodor had the same father, their respective afflictions were genetic through the paternal side. Although Peter's epilepsy was symptomatically of the acquired type, basically it probably was not of that order. Acquired epilepsy occurs three times as often among persons whose heredity disposes them to epileptic attacks as it does among persons of non-epileptic lineage. We may say then that acquired epilepsy is usually "triggered" by hereditary epilepsy, needing only an appropriate incident to set off the explosive discharge.

Accounts state that Peter was "always shaking his head and grimacing, and his right arm was never still." The constant head-shaking and jerking of the arm are characteristic of *epilepsia partialis continua*, that is, continuing small localized motor seizures. At times his head shook worse than at other times and his right arm "flapped like the wing of a crippled bird." It appears that the spells usually stopped there, but sometimes they "marched on" to become generalized convulsions. In the latter case they probably recurred at short intervals, for it is stated that he was occasionally disabled for as long as two weeks at a time. It is evident that he suffered from a focal disturbance on or near the surface of the brain in a motor zone. It is possible that modern neurosurgery could have done much for Peter.

In 1685, Peter had smallpox and lay in a prolonged delirium. His life was despaired of, but the patriarch prayed so hard that Heaven, which had intended to claim the boy, finally relented and granted him a new destiny. Peter awakened suddenly and asked for news of all that had happened during his lapse of consciousness.

His sister Sophia enjoyed her power as regent, but the people did not believe in women rulers and were constantly talking about the day when Peter should become old enough to take the throne. The only way Sophia could make her position secure was to eliminate both Ivan and Peter. The temptation was irresistible, and she began to consider methods for the destruction of the two heirs. Her lover, Vasil Galitzen, one of the three or four best scholars in Russia and a man of humane instincts, opposed any such measures. Boris Galitzen, cousin of Vasil, may have learned of the plot from the latter. At any rate, Boris liked Peter and detested Sophia, and he brought Peter the first news of his sister's plans. The boy was incredulous, but Boris kept repeating the warnings until eventually Peter's fears and anger were aroused. At the annual celebration of the taking of Kazan he sought out Sophia and confronted her with evidence of her murderous ambition. Startled, she made no denial. Finally Peter said bluntly: "Your regency is at an end. Get out!"

Sophia disdained to obey her brother's command, placing her faith in the fickle Streltzy, and Peter fled terror-stricken. His faithful *poteshny*, however, rallied to his side and was strengthened by increasing numbers of the Streltzy who were deserting Sophia's cause. Peter, now seventeen, manfully conquered his panic, if not his fear, and sent his army against the palace. The strength of the attacking force was augmented on the way and the mission was quickly completed. Sophia was seized, deposited in a nunnery, and ordered to stay there or die. As it turned out, she did both. Peter had remained discreetly behind until the army could attain its objectives and prepare the palace for his reception. He then returned to Moscow in triumph and was hailed as czar by the nation. After the celebrations of his accession were ended and proper vengeance had been taken on Sophia's fellow conspirators, he enjoyed official life but briefly. Affairs of state were irksome and the continual round of social functions a complete bore. He craved physical activity and honest comradeship. In consequence, he turned the rule of the country over to his mother's family, the

Narishkins, and betook himself back to his beloved Peobrajensky to occupy his time with soldiering, carpentering, and two new pursuits learned from foreigners, namely, shipbuilding and the manufacture of fireworks.

On January 28, 1689, about six months before Sophia was ousted from the regency, Peter had yielded to his mother's solicitations and taken a bride. She was the beautiful Eudoxia Lopuhkin, who came of a wealthy family and was said to be "endowed with a wealth of piety and good sense." Apparently in the Russia of that time it was not believed that piety and good sense are irreconcilable!

Eudoxia was three years older than Peter, but since he was being married to please his mother, the difference in age was more her concern than his. Three days after the wedding he had another one of his "spells" and was carried to his bed. He recovered quickly, however, and was soon able to join in the wedding celebration which his enforced absence had in no wise interrupted. He sought out his beloved *poteshny* and proceeded to outdrink the best and the worst of them. After about two and one-half months of married life, he left his home and Eudoxia and sped to Lake Pereslavl eager to see how his shipbuilding was proceeding. Once there he filled his stomach with vodka, rolled up his sleeves, seized his hammer, and went to work. After six weeks he returned to his bride and his mother only because the latter had deputed Tiphon Streshniev to bring him back by using whatever force was necessary. Eudoxia greeted her returned husband delightedly. He kissed her and then hurried off for a round of drinks with his *poteshny*.

Just outside Preobrajensky was a colony of several thousand foreigners. A few of Wallenstein's defeated troopers and some Englishmen had founded the colony of Sloboda, as it was known, but not until the arrival of some three thousand Scottish adventurers did the place acquire an aspect of prosperity and permanence. To these early settlers were added business intermediaries with wives and families, so that by the year 1700 all the states of western Europe were represented. Peter made the acquaintance of one of the Scots, a huge fellow with a jovial manner, an unquenchable thirst, and a head full of useful information. He could speak Russian fluently and identified himself as General Patrick Gordon. Being a citizen of the Sloboda, he was a royalist Roman catholic and as such was anathema to the Patriarchate; nevertheless, he and Peter became fast friends and Gordon accepted Peter's invitations to dine at the Kremlin. Joachim, the Pontiff, was outraged and ordered the practice stopped. Although Peter did not dare disobey the holy command, he expressed to Gordon his detestation of the priest. Shortly, Joachim died. Peter did not invite Gordon to the Kremlin again but, instead, went to Sloboda himself and dined with the General. The young Czar, who had never been in Sloboda before, was amazed at the order and cleanliness he saw there. The attractive gardens, the neatly kept squares, and the trees, flowers, and fountains seemed to him inexpressibly beautiful. The manners and customs of the people were different, too. At dinner they did not wipe their mouths with the backs of their hands or the tablecloth, and they did not throw chicken bones and other food refuse on the floor. Their women dressed much more attractively than the Russian women, mingled freely with the men, and seemed very intelligent. He danced with them, and as his fingers pressed against their whalebone corsets, he marveled at the firmness of their bodies. There was one unavoidable conclusion to be drawn from his observations at Sloboda—the foreigners were infinitely superior to the Russians, who were a nation of ignorant, hide-bound Asiatics. Peter fixed his eyes on western Europe and became a confirmed Xenophil. This obsession gave him the strength to lift the great Russian nation out of barbarism and into the society of European peoples.

In addition to Gordon there was another man whom Peter met at Sloboda, a Swiss named Lefort, who became a dependable friend and counselor. Lefort was a handsome, well-educated man, nearly as tall as Peter and even more powerful physically. Like Gordon he was skilled in the use of arms and was made a general in the army of the Czar. Probably neither of these men had much to do with the shaping of Peter's policies of government, but they trained armies for him and sometimes restrained him in his moments of drunken rashness when no one else dared to interfere. In February, 1690, Eudoxia gave birth to a son. The father, who had almost forgotten that he had a wife, went into transports of joy. He hugged and kissed Eudoxia, proclaimed a period of public rejoicing, gave a splendid display of fireworks, and got drunk. He was a man now and strong drink was the gift of the gods to men. He would drink a toast to the gods of drink, a form of worship in which he showed himself to be surpassingly devout.

The natal celebrations ended, Peter quickly lost interest in both Eudoxia and Alexis, the son. He had never cared for his wife anyhow. Wives were a nuisance, though perhaps a necessary nuisance if a Czar was to have a direct heir. But wives were forever making demands, while other women, of whom there was always a sufficient abundance, were sheer enjoyment. A man could take them and then kick them out after he'd had enough of them. So Peter perferred not to bother with Eudoxia or to be bothered by her. The confounded priests were always getting between him and his pleasure, too, but he would bide his time and take care of them when the opportunity came. He wanted freedom and he would have no women or effeminate monks telling him what to do or how to do it. So he went his way, making love to the wives and mistresses of his friends and any other desirable women who crossed his path. Sometimes he had sex frenzies when neither beauty nor femaleness mattered. And always, at intervals, would come the spells. In his maturity they seemed somewhat different from those that he suffered during his adolescence. They were characterized by only minor convulsive movements, but there was an overpowering sense of fear, his mind was dull, he manifested a peculiar credulousness in which he took common figures of speech literally, and he was fit for neither work nor play. Wine and vodka, the natural antidotes for depressed spirits, seemed only to delay recovery.

To lighten his moods and to ridicule the priests and others whom he hated but dared not touch, Peter organized the Council of High Buffoonery. When the Council held a masquerade, he marched at the head of the procession carrying a large drum which he beat thunderously. His fellow actors were drawn from the *poteshny* and the troop of twenty-five to thirty dwarfs which he maintained in the vicinity of the palace. Frederick William of Prussia, who was five feet, four inches in height, had his Potsdam giants; his friend Peter of Russia, who was six feet, seven inches had his midgets. The one wished to look up, the other to look down.

Peter's sense of humor, it would seem, took grotesque turns. Voltaire thought the burlesques on the priesthood masterpieces of satire. However, since Voltaire was himself a satirist and a hater of priests, it is unlikely that his usual critical judgment was without bias on this point. There is a description of one of the conclaves of the Council which was held at what was termed the Vaticanium, the home of the old tutor Zutov, who was dubbed "Prince Pope." First of all, four attendants escorted the Elect, clad in the red robe of a cardinal, into the hall of the consistory where he mounted a throne made of barrels decorated with bottles and drinking glasses. At the head of a procession came Peter dressed as a Dutch sailor and beating a drum. Zutov followed astride a hogshead drawn by four oxen and surrounded by mimic monks. These were followed in turn by carts drawn by pigs, goats, elk, and bears. The "cells" of the audience members were casks sawed in two, one half for food and drink and the other half for the natural residue of digestion. For the delectation of all, there was a notorious strumpet dressed as a "Princess-Abbess." For such theatrical carousals Peter would plan for days with the expenditure of much time and money.

Other programs devised by Peter were so fantastically pointless as to be worthy only of a disordered mind. For example, on one occasion he invited some foreign envoys, soaked and miserable after a trip at sea, to come to Peterhof for a drinking party. After the party the envoys, who were given no opportunity to dry their clothes, were compelled to sleep half-frozen in the open. At four A.M. their host roused them, gave each man an axe, and bade them all follow him to a grove where they were ordered to cut an alley from one side of the wood to the other. Having finished their task at seven o'clock, they were solemnly thanked by Peter for their co-operation and commanded to return to the palace for the evening. At the appointed hour and place the guests were regaled with much liquor and sent to bed. At midnight they were called and made to go to the room of the newly wed Prince of Circassia, who was in bed with his wife. Orders were for them to stay the night in the nuptial chamber emptying bottles. At eight

A.M., they were notified to go to the castle for breakfast. There they were shown how to swallow a glass of vodka at one gulp, and each man was require to demonstrate his mastery of the technique. Next they were sent to a high hill to take the air, and then to the bottom of the hill where a peasant with eight miserable nags without saddles awaited them. Each guest was ordered to mount and in comic array, the party paraded before the Emperor-host who reviewed them from a bedroom window with his arms propped on a sill. It has been suggested that Peter may have wished to humiliate the envoys, or, perhaps, he found enjoyment in appearing to confirm rumors of his insanity. At any rate, we should credit him with a contribution to our modern system of education, since he undoubtedly set the pattern for the initiation rites for some of today's college fraternities.

During his first tour of the western European countries Peter took lessons in anatomy at Leyden and, as a result, fancied himself something of a dentist and surgeon. He delighted in pulling teeth, and he also essayed to perform a few surgical operations. On one occasion he tapped the abdomen of an elderly woman who suffered from dropsy and withdrew a large quantity of fluid. The patient expired a few days later and the Czar-surgeon, very considerately, attended her funeral. In 1715 the Czarina, Martha, died. Peter had long been curious to know whether the girl who had been married to his moribund brother, Feodor, was actually the model of virtue she was reputed to be. He made a post-mortem examination of the body and was immensely pleased to find physical evidence of her fidelity to the long-dead Czar. In 1706 Peter founded the first military hospital in Moscow and staffed it with surgeons brought from Paris. Soon after he opened a school of surgery with his French military surgeons acting as instructors.

While Peter was nearing the city of Vienna on the return from his historic trip to the west countries of Europe, he received news of a revolt among the troublesome Streltzy. He hastened home, the personification of fury, and decreed the penalty of extinction not only for the organization but for its individual members as well. For days on end he labored joyously, wielding with his own powerful arms the axe or the sword against the necks of the traitorous members.

The son, Alexis, was a great disappointment to his father. Far from being interested in the arts and sciences of war, he was a pious weakling who for all his piety was a confirmed drunkard, a beast of a husband and, what Peter abhorred most, a coward and an ignoramus. The Czar greatly desired his son's assistance in the crucial war against the Swedes, but the recreant Czarevitch with his Finnish mistress hid in various cities of Europe for months before he was found and lured back to the Fatherland. There he was brought to trial on a charge of traitorous conduct and, at his father's insistence, sentenced to death. Characteristically, Peter declared: "I have not spared myself or my soldiers! I shall not spare my son." Then one morning Alexis was reportedly found dead in his prison cell. The cause of his demise was officially stated to have been apoplexy brought on by the shock of hearing his death sentence. It is generally believed, however, that he succumbed to poison or to violence.

Peter repudiated his marriage to Eudoxia shortly after the birth of Alexis because allegedly she gave encouragement to the reactionary party. In 1706 he was married privately to a buxom young Livonian woman who had been a maid-servant to the Lutheran Pastor Gluck, of Marienburg, and then mistress in turn to Generals Sheremetov and Menschikov. She was known by the name of Catherine. Peter had a veritable harem at the time of his marriage to Catherine, but he liked to have her with him because her presence seemed to calm him. Sometimes when he felt a spell coming on, he could bury his head in her ample bosom and quickly regain his composure. Subsequently, in order to qualify her for possible succession to the throne, he was married to her in public.

Peter is commonly believed to have had syphilis, and it would seem that no person with his utterly promiscuous sexual habits could escape the disease. A French chronicler records that while at Amsterdam the Czar had suffered "a disgrace in the courts of love." He was given courses of treatment with mercury in 1706 as well as in 1707 and 1708, and his physicians made no secret of the fact that he was suffering from a venereal disease. These records of venereal infection treated with mercury do not in themselves, however, constitute reliable evidence that Peter had syphilis, for at that time only one venereal disease was recognized. The hard

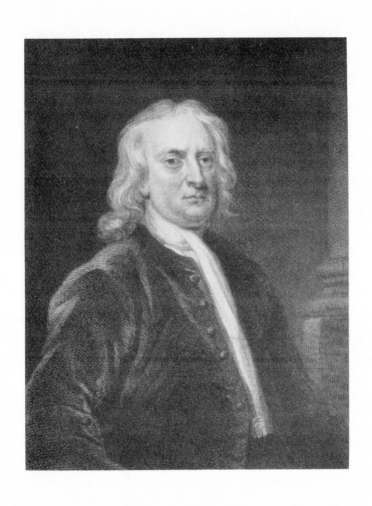

SIR ISAAC NEWTON

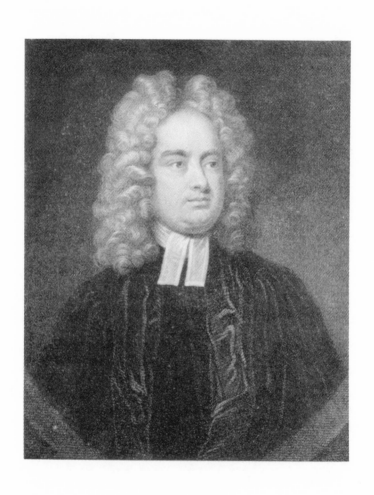

DEAN SWIFT

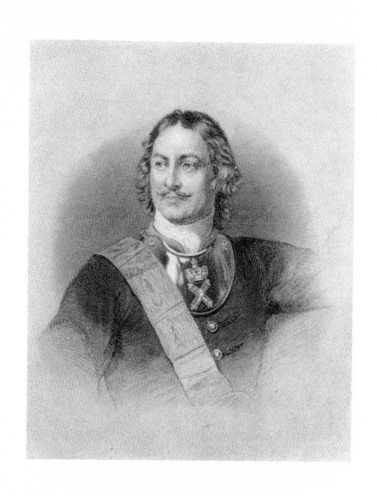

PETER THE GREAT

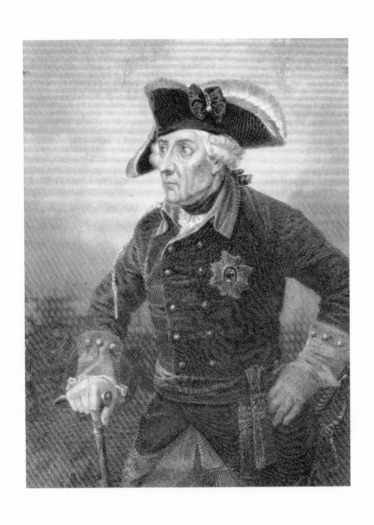

FREDERICK THE GREAT

chancre, the soft chancre, and the purulent discharge of gonorrhoea were all thought to be manifestations of a single disease,
syphilis, and hence were accorded the same treatment. There is
some clinical evidence that he had *tabes dorsalis*, a late syphilitic
involvement of the spinal cord characterized especially by lan-
cinating pains of the lower extremities and even today commonly
mistaken for rheumatism by those unskilled in diagnosis. As he
was said to have had rheumatism in the last two decades of his life
and to have suffered excruciating pain, it seems probable that
Peter actually had *tabes*.

In 1716 he suffered a sudden attack of paralysis of one arm,
but a very skillfully applied wooden splint enabled him to use the
member to an increasing extent so that eventually he was able to
remove the support and to use the arm as well as ever. This episode
may have been the result of vascular syphilis involving one of the
motor areas of the brain. More likely, however, since it ended in
complete recovery, it was a "Saturday night palsy," a pressure
paralysis of the musculospiral nerve resulting in wrist drop. This
condition is especially likely to occur in persons who, in the stupor
of drunkenness, either sit with an arm hanging over the back of a
chair or lie with it dangling over the side of a bed. A certain amount
of circumstantial evidence that Peter had syphilis is found in the
fact that the disease is known to have been rampant not only in
Amsterdam but in all the seaports where he sojourned and, of
course, caroused in the course of his western tour.

During the last ten years of his life, the state of Peter's health
was one of irregular decline. He had frequent severe attacks of
bronchitis and subsequently suffered equally severe attacks of
asthma whenever he caught a cold. In 1721 he became moody,
went into frequent tantrums, suffered from headache and insomnia, and never stopped grimacing and shaking his head. At
night he saw ghosts and streams of blood. He suffered from a constant desire to urinate. Undoubtedly his bladder was overfull and
as a result of "back pressure" on the kidneys he was slightly uremic.
The obstructive symptoms were possibly due to stricture resulting
from gonorrhoea, though they may have been caused by bladder
stone, or prostatic disease or syphilitic involvement of the nerves
controlling bladder function. Finally the urine dribbled more free-

ly and he felt better. In 1722 his trouble was better and worse by turns, but the next year he was bedfast a great deal of the time. In the late summer of 1724 his doctors diagnosed an attack of gravel complicated by a venereal disorder which had been badly cared for. He is said to have passed a sizable stone, aided by the doctor's probings, after which his bladder function was much improved, though his thighs and groin were covered with open sores—likely the result of skin irritation and infection due to clothes constantly wet with urine.

In October, Peter proclaimed himself cured and declared that he had never felt better in all his life. Then, fitting the deed to the word, he set out for Lake Ladoga and rode horseback for many miles through the frozen marshes to see what progress was being made with the canal works in that area. On the return journey he saw a boat aground and its crew in peril near the village of Lahta. With characteristic rashness, he plunged waist-deep into the ice cold water and helped to rescue the crew. By the time he reached St. Petersburg, on November 2, he was feverish and ready for the sick-bed. Two days later he was on his feet again. Next day he was informed by the secret chancery that Catherine had taken as lover a William Mons, brother of Peter's first mistress, Anna Mons. Peter was thunderstruck. For two weeks he took counsel with himself. Then he had Mons arrested and condemned for accepting bribes—the presents which outsiders had given him as the price of intercessions with Catherine for petty business and social favors. On the morning of November 28, Mons was led to his doom.

Catherine confessed a fondness for Mons and admitted having given him a gold ring, but that was all. Her manner was so forthright and her statements so plausible that many, including some influential senators, expressed doubt of her guilt. She waited calmly for Peter to make up his mind. He let his intimates know that he intended to administer to her the same punishment that had been meted out to William Mons. France, it so happened, was destined to save her. Peter was hoping to marry his favorite and most favored daughter, Elizabeth, to Louis XV. The French diplomat, Campredon, informed the Czar that the marriage would be quite impossible if the girl's mother were to be executed, so Peter decided to wait.

On January 9, 1725, he took to his bed with a recurrence of his old ailment. His bladder was enormously distended, he could pass almost no urine, and his suffering was intense. As he lay in agony, he is said to have exclaimed, "What a wretched animal is man!" After two weeks a "tapping operation" was done on the advice of an Italian surgeon named Lazoretti. This operation consisted of forcing a hollow needle through the wall of the lower abdomen and into the cavity of the greatly distended bladder. The relief was immediate, but the respite was brief. The patient continued to grow weaker. He called for Prakopovitch, bishop of Pskov, confessed his sins and received the sacrament. On January 27, several hours after the senators had assured Catherine of her succession, Peter called for a pencil and paper. He traced out the barely legible words, "Give everything back to——" There his hand relaxed and the pencil fell from his grasp. He was unable to finish his last will and testament. At an early hour the next morning he died.

The immediate cause of Peter's death was urinary obstruction with infection of the bladder, kidneys, and accessory organs. He did very well indeed to live nearly fifty-three years.

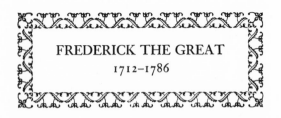

FREDERICK THE GREAT
1712–1786

Iꜰ Fʀᴇᴅᴇʀɪᴄᴋ Wɪʟʟɪᴀᴍ I, father of Frederick the Great of Prussia, possessed a single laudable trait of character it seems that his biographers have been unable to discover it. With truly remarkable unanimity he is described as having been a brutal bully, unclean in mind and body, scornful of gentility and the arts, and niggardly in everything not pertaining to his army. He loved his army more than he loved his gold. He compelled his family to live on coarse vegetables and the cheapest of foods, and if they dared complain of their diet he threw pewter plates at their heads. But to secure recruits for his regiment of Potsdam giants, he spent vast sums and, quite incidentally, assembled the finest collection of cases of hyperpituitarism ever heard of.

Frederick William's single social indulgence was his *Tobaks Kollegium* where he habitually spent his evenings drinking beer, smoking, and exchanging coarse gossip with his intimates. Some of his associates were *Junkers* whom he distrusted; the others were substantial burghers of whose complete personal loyalty he was assured. His court reflected the vulgarity and parsimony of its master. And with all this, the King, having no sense of the ridiculous, was fanatically religious. Thus was born the "*Gott und Ich*" complex which in the House of Hohenzollern was seemingly to take on genetic attributes. At times Frederick William's religious fervor was so intense and his devotions so prolonged that his family and servants were unable to keep up with him and became physically, and probably also spiritually, exhausted.

Such was the setting into which Fate, by the processes of nature, dropped the frail and sensitive little Frederick, the fourth of fourteen children born of the marriage of Frederick William I and his cousin, Sophie Dorothea, of Hanover. Of the fourteen, ten survived infancy. For the first seven years of his life Frederick was under the direct care of Madame de Roucoulles, who in turn was responsible to an "honorary governess," Frau von Kamecke. Madame Roucoulles, who had also been Frederick William's nurse, was devoted and kind. But for her tender watchfulness Frederick might well have gone the way of his two elder brothers who perished in their babyhood.

As a child, Frederick was abnormally small for his age, delicate, shy, and nervous. He jumped at unexpected noises and pulled the bed covers over his head in the dark. Of his brothers and sisters he cared only for Wilhelmine. She was several years older than Frederick, towards whom she adopted a protective attitude. To the end of their days Frederick and Wilhelmine lived in adoration of each other.

To Frederick William his little son was a great disappointment. "Never perhaps in all the history of the world," wrote Voltaire, "have a father and son ever existed who were quite so unlike." The child, totally unable to comprehend the parent's rude manner and blustering talk, responded with a wide-eyed terrified silence. When the King raised his voice, as he invariably did, in an effort to scold an answer out of little Frederick, the only response he elicited was a fearful shaking of the thin little body. Many years later Wilhelmine wrote, "The King could not bear my brother; he abused him whenever he laid eyes on him so that Frederick became obsessed with a fear of him which persisted after the age of reason." Because German was the language of his father, Frederick always held that tongue in detestation. With his nurse and his sister Wilhelmine he invariably conversed in French; when he was required to use German, he spoke or wrote it incorrectly.

Frederick William was determined to make a soldier, in his opinion the only sort of man worthwhile, out of Frederick. When the child had attained the age of five years, he was rigged out in

73

the uniform of a noncommissioned officer of the Prussian Army and supplied with a small drum. He cried in resentment against the cumbrous clothes, but to his father's momentary delight he beat the drum vigorously. On his seventh birthday Frederick was taken from the custody of his female nurses and handed over to three male tutors. Two of these were army officers, General Count von Finkenstein and Colonel von Kalkstein, and their task was to inculcate military virtues and love of the army on the tiny Crown Prince. A young Frenchman, Jacques Egide Duhan de Jandun, commonly known as Duhan, was chosen to attend to Frederick's formal education. Had the King known more of Duhan, he would not have entrusted Frederick to his care. The Frenchman was a man of refined tastes and democratic instincts and he was an excellent pedagogue. Moreover, he loved Frederick and rejoiced at the progress made by his royal pupil. Soon after Duhan's appointment he and General Finkenstein took their charge to Wusterhausen, a quiet country place near Berlin, for moral, military, and mental training of the peculiar type deemed most suitable for a future king of Prussia. To begin with, there were certain basic objectives to be achieved. First of all, Frederick "must be so thoroughly informed as to God's omnipotence that he will always have a holy fear and veneration for his creator." Then he was to be taught to "revere, esteem, and obey" his parents; finally, and most wonderfully of all, he was to feel "true love and perfect confidence towards his father."

The routine which the King prescribed for Frederick and which was enforced for more than nine years allowed very little time for childish recreation and only seven and one-half hours out of the twenty-four for sleep. With almost no games or exercises in the open air, a diet completely unsuitable for a child, and an ogre for a father, it is not surprising that Frederick's adolescence brought neither stability of the nervous system nor greatly increased bodily vigor. The frail child became a weak, spindly-legged, nervous youth who shunned normal physical activity, caught cold easily, and suffered frequent severe attacks of indigestion. His hatred for his father remained undiminished. Each visit by the King meant an aftermath of belly-ache for Frederick.

Between the King's frequent visits Duhan surreptitiously instructed his pupil in Latin and the classics, subjects for which the young Prince showed a strong predilection. Another extracurricular activity consisted in lessons on the flute. We can easily believe that Frederick quickly attained a proficiency which fully explored the musical potentialities of that instrument. But eventually Duhan incurred the displeasure of the King and was summarily dismissed. Thereafter Frederick wrote his beloved tutor that when he came into his own money Duhan should receive a pension of twenty-four hundred crowns annually. The promise was fulfilled.

Late in the year 1727, Frederick William had an attack of religion of such unwonted intensity that the integrity of the state was imperiled. Shrewd Baron Grumkow, who was the King's most trusted adviser, urged a trip to Dresden for a visit with Augustus the Strong, king of Saxony and Poland, who had his court in that city. No better choice could possibly have been made for a man who needed to lose an excess of piety. Return to normalcy was signalized after a fortnight when Frederick William forsook the Holy Ghost and took himself a mistress.

Young Frederick would have been glad to go to Dresden even in company with his father, but the latter would hear nothing of it. Wilhelmine, however, knew how to pull the right strings and shortly after Frederick William's arrival in Dresden, Augustus requested him to send for the Crown Prince. The Prussian King could hardly refuse his host's request, and Frederick, who had just turned sixteen, had the time of his life. It is said that Augustus and Grumkow kept the King occupied so that the youngster was fairly free of paternal supervision. But it is a fair guess that neither father nor son wanted the other to know all that was going on.

After Frederick's return to Berlin he found the old routine of life unbearably dull and onerous. He was mentally depressed and physically exhausted. The King was notified that his heir-apparent was suffering from "a lingering fever" and was "threatened with [a diagnosis of] tuberculosis." Because of his indisposition Frederick was relieved of some of his most arduous military duties, but Frederick William, who hated any sort of weakness, bullied and nagged the boy more than ever. In May, 1728, Augustus came to Berlin to repay Frederick William's visit to Dresden, bringing with him the young Countess Orczelska whom Frederick had greatly admired during his sojourn at the court of Augustus. The Countess was very gracious toward Frederick with the result that his health improved astonishingly during the few weeks she was at Potsdam. But when the visitors had gone, his life seemed harder than ever before and more than ever he resented his father's bullying.

He sought emotional release in an unseemly friendship with one of his father's pages, a youth named Keith. When the King learned of the attachment, he was furious. Frederick was sent to Wusterhausen to repent of his sin and Keith was expelled from the court and sent to an army camp near the Dutch frontier. After a few days at Wusterhausen Frederick wrote his father a bootlicking letter of apology which was rejected by the addressee in language both plain and forceful. After several weeks in a sort of moral quarantine the Prince was permitted to return to Berlin, where he promptly entered into a "love" affair with a young Prussian army captain who was about six years his senior. The captain, whose name was Hans Herman von Katte, had been educated as a lawyer and was, by Wilhelmine's admission, "well read and intelligent." Katte hated Frederick William and the Prussian military system, and he missed no opportunity to help Frederick evade the tyrannous regime imposed by his father. He was glad, therefore, for reasons both worthy and unworthy, to arrange a secret loan for the Prince by a large banking firm in Berlin so that he might buy a small library of the works of Descartes, Voltaire, Locke, and other philosophers. After the books were purchased, they were hidden in the home of a friendly Berlin merchant. Somehow Frederick William learned of Frederick's debts and had the boy brought before him. In a most terrible access of fury he attacked the Prince with his fists and might have beaten him to death had not a courageous valet interposed to drag the hapless lad beyond the reach of his maddened parent. This episode determined Frederick to run away from home regardless of any peril such a venture might entail.

What seemed a favorable opportunity for escape presented itself. The King was planning a journey which would bring him to Wesel on the Dutch frontier. Frederick was to accompany his father, and according to a scheme worked out by Katte, the harrassed Prince would, at the proper moment, cross the line into

Holland, proceed to The Hague where he would meet Katte, and thence to London and the protection of his uncle, King George II. Unfortunately Frederick lost his head completely, bungled the execution of the plan, and was arrested by royal command as an army deserter. Katte's complicity was revealed by a misdirected letter written by Frederick. Both the conspirators were imprisoned in the fortress of Kustrin near Berlin. Katte was tried by court-martial and sentenced to three years imprisonment, but Frederick William overruled the action of the military court and had the captain beheaded just below the window of Frederick's cell. The shock which resulted from witnessing the death of Katte threw Frederick into a faint followed by a strange attitude of dazed in-difference. Gradually, however, his emotional and intellectual patterns returned to their norms, thanks to the merciful haze of unreality which envelops tragic experiences when viewed in retro-spect and protects the mind against continued trauma to itself.

The inner nature of Frederick's affairs with Keith and Katte is, of course, not certainly known, but the implications of homo-sexuality are overwhelming. Only during his sojourn at the court of Augustus and the months immediately following did Frederick manifest any interest in women. In his early maturity he wrote, "I love the fair sex but my love is unstable. I want only to enjoy women. . . . I despise them afterwards." In 1733 he was married by royal command to Princess Elisabeth Christine, niece of the Em-press of Austria. Frederick did his best to wriggle out of the match, but the King was adamant as usual and the wedding was celebrated at the appointed time and place. On the night of the wedding day the Prince sent his wife to her apartments while he retired to his own. He continued to live apart from her, and he always insisted that the union had never been consummated. For the rest of his life Frederick treated her with formal politeness and at no time, so far as anyone knows, did he manifest the slightest affection for her or even the least personal interest in her.

It is true that at one time Frederick was known to be calling quite regularly on the wife of his Colonel, Frau von Wreech, a charming and accomplished lady, but his biographers agree, some of them rather regretfully, that his relations with her were emi-nently correct. Hegemann credits Dr. Ritter von Zimmermann,

77

one-time physician to both Frederick William and Frederick, with the assertion that the latter "contracted a venereal disease shortly before his betrothal" and that complications of so dire a nature ensued that castration was performed before cure was effected. If von Zimmermann's allegation is true, it means that Frederick probably had gonorrhoea complicated by double epididymitis, for the relief of which both testicles were removed—heroic treatment, indeed, but not unheard of in the medicine of Frederick's time. It happens, however, that Dr. von Zimmermann had such a poor reputation for veracity that his statements are not to be given full credence. It is possible, of course, that only one testicle was removed (unilateral orchidectomy). If this was done, the endocrine effects would be inconsequential; the psychic effects would depend upon what the patient expected or thought of his operation. But it must be said that even a simple gonorrheal epididymitis, without the added penalty of surgery, is a painful experience, the remembrance of which might conceivably make a woman-hater out of a theretofore normally philogynous male.

After the Katte affair Frederick's spirit seemed completely broken. He recovered his composure, but all thought of escape from his father and the system his father had created was abandoned. The King assigned him to the Civil Service in Kustrin for instruction in agriculture, finance, and trade. To the surprise of everyone he settled down to his work manfully, displaying unsuspected mental keenness and administrative ability. He now had his own household and a small allowance for his personal needs. In his hours of leisure he studied music, read enormously, and tried his hand at writing poetry. At the age of eighteen he had begun to find himself intellectually. But he had no real companionship in Kustrin and he longed for fellowship with kindred spirits. The first and most difficult step would be to convince Frederick William that his wayward son was truly penitent and the watchwords of his amendment were filial love and obedience.

Frederick wrote scores of letters in which he abjectly begged forgiveness and hypocritically protested his love for his tormentor. When his father came to visit him in August, 1731, Frederick's books were hidden, his household was in order, and his attitude was one of respectful obedience. The King was favorably impressed though by no means convinced. During the ensuing months, however, reports of Frederick's conduct were so satisfactory that the King was moved to commission him colonel of a regiment quartered at Ruppin, which became his official place of residence for the next eight years. It was during his first year at Ruppin that Frederick's enforced marriage to Princess Elisabeth Christine occurred.

Although his behavior toward Frederick William was that of servile adoration, Frederick confessed that his hatred of the King was as great as ever and that he was merely marking time until his oppressor should die, "for after all," he said to Wilhelmine, "I realize that I shall experience no good days as long as he lives."

As early as 1734 Frederick William had shown evidence of failing circulation and in the next six years his ailment was characterized by several dropsical episodes. The dropsy subsided with rest and medical care, but the disease marched on and the King was compelled to curb his physical activity between times also. Meanwhile Frederick had taken up his residence at Rheinsberg in the country house his father had given him for a wedding present. The ailing King complained occasionally about his son's indolence, but he lacked the energy to interfere seriously with his manner of life. For the first time Frederick was free to live as he chose. In a strictly masculine household he surrounded himself with artists, scientists, and scholars of literature. It was at this time that he began his correspondence with Voltaire engendering a friendship which, though full of contradictions, was nevertheless genuine and lasting.

In June, 1740, after a year and a half of continuous confinement for Frederick William, his tough old heart beat its last systole. Frederick had been constrained to spend many weeks at his father's side during the final period of invalidism, and the experience was a trying one indeed. The King, though coughing and gasping for breath, raged at Frederick by the hour. Possibly Frederick's consolation was the obvious fact that Frederick William's exertions were hastening the approach of the end. The strain of it all, however, was affecting Frederick's health. He lost considerable weight and on one occasion suffered an attack of intestinal cramps, probably a nervous manifestation, which alarmed his doctors greatly.

Upon Frederick's accession to the throne his ministers, who had expected to run the government to suit themselves, received the shock of their lives. He discharged some of them and defined the duties of the others, making all subservient, at all times, to his will. He even donned a stiff Prussian uniform and took command of the army. The court was amazed at his industry. His rule was both more autocratic and more refined than that of his father. The Giant Guards regiment was abolished at once; his old friend Keith was made a lieutenant colonel and given a post in Berlin; and August William, the new King's younger brother, was designated prince of Prussia and heir to the throne. He lifted the censorship from newspapers and pleased the common people by proclaiming complete religious freedom.

In the first months of his reign he made a grand tour of the country to receive the homage of his subjects and, more importantly, to have his first meeting with Voltaire, whom he literally worshiped. It is said that on his way to this meeting Frederick was stricken with a fever, but it seems more likely that he was actually prostrated with excitement at the prospect of coming face to face with his idol. When Voltaire arrived at the Castle of Meuse, where the King's journey had been interrupted by illness, the famous Frenchman was led into his Majesty's private chamber. "By the light of a candle," writes Voltaire, "I saw a miserable little cot . . . on which lay a little man dressed in a ridiculous dressing gown made of heavy blue coth. This was the King, who was perspiring and trembling under an inadequate cover in an attack of fever. I bowed and began our acquaintance by feeling his pulse as though I were his chief physician. The attack passed. He arose and came to the table. Algarotti, Keyserlingk, his secretary—we all had supper together and discussed at length the immortality of the soul, freedom, and Plato's hermaphrodites." So ended, apparently, King Frederick's "fever." But release from the tyranny of the old King did not cure Frederick's neuroticism. In the year of his accession he complained to Dr. Eller, his court physician, that he was "more sensitive" about his health and he wished to have remedies at hand for every possible illness.

His desire to prove that his sense of inferiority was not well founded may have induced Frederick to undertake the sudden invasion of Silesia which began his war with Austria. When he saw that his generalship had failed at Mollwitz, his first important battle, he fled the field, leaving the war in the laps of his generals. When messengers caught up with him to apprise him of "his" victory, he was cowering in an old mill near the town of Oppeln in a condition bordering on hysteria. But Frederick possessed the basic methodicalness of his race. Immediately he set about analyzing his battle tactics to discover where and how he had erred in order to avoid a repetition of his mistakes. The successive victories of Hohenfriedberg, Soor, and Kesseldorf established his military reputation beyond question and upon his return to Berlin he was everywhere called "Frederick the Great."

As he approached middle age King Frederick began to complain of painful joints in his hands aggravated by grasping the reins as he rode his horse. His physicians are said to have called the condition "gout," but as it appears to have involved the hands alone, it seems likely that the disease was what is now known as Heberden's nodes, a type of osteoarthritis affecting the bases of the terminal phalanges of the fingers of both hands and often attended by considerable soreness with permanent deformity and some degree of disability. The cause and cure of the disorder are unknown, but its image is now in the medical spectrum and analysis must follow betimes.

At a time of life when most men would incline toward less work, Frederick inclined toward more work. He labored with machinelike precision and indefatigability. In summer he arose at three o'clock and in winter at four, regardless of how late he had been up the previous night. He dressed without concern for appearances or even cleanliness. He was careful of what he ate because of his weak digestion, but enjoyed his food nonetheless. A competent allergist could have helped his Majesty a great deal in the problem of selecting his diet.

After he took up his residence at Sans Souci, he demanded stimulating conversation at the dinner table and often spent the evening playing the flute or discussing art and literature with his intimates. It was said that Sans Souci was a "mixture of Athens and

81

Sparta" where the King "acted Mars all morning and played the role of Apollo in the evening." There were no Germans in Frederick's social clique and the French language was always the medium of conversation. All women were *personae non gratae* at Sans Souci. Frederick had become a complete misogynist if, indeed, he was not always such. His sister Wilhelmine was the only woman for whom he felt any love or admiration and that, he said, was because she had the mind of a man.

With battle experience he became indifferent to danger, not hesitating to enter the thickest of the fight. In one hot skirmish during the Seven Years' War he had three horses shot from under him, but he came through the war unscathed. When on a campaign his mania for writing verse was more pronounced than ever. It became his habit to compose a few stanzas each night in order to make his mind more receptive to sleep. If, however, the war was not going well for him, nothing could calm him and his health became wretched. At such times his belly seemed to harbor a battleground on which his digestion and his food waged constant warfare against each other. At the end of the Seven Years' War he was, in his own words, "old, broken, grayhaired, wrinkled." But if he looked aged and shrunken, his eyes were as piercing as ever and his intellect still razor-edged. The conflagration which had been set off inside him by assumption of his kingly role flamed as fiercely as ever. "I have infinite infirmities and illnesses," he wrote Voltaire, "and I cure myself with hard work and patience." The reconstruction of Prussia after the war offered a task difficult enough to absorb all the energy he could give to it. But despite his assertions to the contrary, neither hard work in pursuits of peace nor the excitement of the battlefield could conquer his ennui.

In his last years Frederick was inclined to review his life with outspoken dissatisfaction. He cursed the insatiable desire for power which had diverted his mind from literary and artistic pursuits. He wished that he might have been a great writer instead of a king; that he might have achieved greatness instead of having greatness thrust upon him.

The first clear break in the health of Frederick came in August, 1785, after he had spent a day in a drenching rain at the Silesian maneuvers. There, it is said, he caught a cold which was followed by an attack of asthma. Though he soon returned to his daily routine of work, he was not well and, it is alleged, suffered a stroke about a month later so that "his physicians did not think he would outlive the day." The correctness of the diagnosis of "stroke" may properly be questioned, for he seems to have returned to his kingly labors a few days after the event with his customary diligence and perspicacity. It was not long, however, before he began to have attacks of asthma following physical exertion in the course of his day's work, and also at night as he rested abed.

Plainly these were attacks of "cardiac asthma" and were due to a failing left ventricle in a heart which was unequal to the task of longer maintaining circulation against the resistance of high blood pressure. With persistent and increasing weakness of the left ventricle, blood was dammed back on the pulmonary side and the right ventricle, too, began to fail. It was then that dropsy ensued and the sick man was completely unable to obtain rest in a recumbent posture. The medical term "orthopnea" is applied to this condition of inability to breathe in any but the upright attitude of body. Concerning this phase of Frederick's illness, Carlyle wrote, "For many months past he has not been in bed but sits day and night in an easy chair, unable to get breath except in that posture."

On August 15, 1786, Frederick did not waken until eleven o'clock in the forenoon and he then seemed confused for some minutes. The next morning his staff of assistants, gathered before the King's chambers, were told to wait—his Majesty was "in a kind of sleep, of stertorous, ominous character." At nine o'clock that night he was coughing in a short, hacking manner and his respiration was becoming more and more difficult. Just after midnight Strutzki, his Kammerhussar, took Frederick's limp but still living body on his knee and for two hours supported the head of the moribund King so that his Highness might not be said to have died of suffocation. On the morning of August 17, 1786, at twenty minutes past the hour of two, Frederick gave his last gasp.

Fittingly enough his body was placed beside that of his father in the Gornison Kirche in Potsdam.[1] Their true memorial, which belongs to one as much as to the other, is found in the wreckage of wars past and in the horror of wars which may come.

[1] According to the *Life* magazine two coffins containing the remains of Frederick and his father, respectively, were found by American soldiers deep in a salt mine in the Thuringian forest near Bernterode on April 27, 1945. Obviously they had been removed from Potsdam to avoid desecration by the advancing Russians. They now lie entombed under the floor of the north transept of St. Elizabeth's Church, Marburg, in the American zone of Germany.

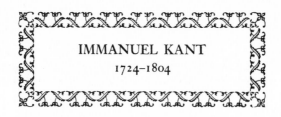

IMMANUEL KANT
1724–1804

ITFREQUENTLY HAPPENS that frail persons, intolerant
of cold, incapable of prolonged muscular exertion, and sensitive
to common articles of diet, may, nevertheless, display a high degree of resistance to disease, perform daily a vast amount of mental
work, and eventually attain a ripe old age. Of that particular bio-
type was Immanuel Kant.

Kant, whose Scottish ancestors spelled the name with a "C"
instead of a "K," was born in Königsburg, Prussia, on April 22,
1724. His parents were of humble rank and of modest means even
for their social station. Immanuel, who was the second of six children, was enabled to secure a liberal education through the help of
a near relative who saw signs of genius in the boy and an outsider
who "esteemed the family for their piety and domestic virtues."
His mother was a woman of exalted character and of intellectual
attainments out of all proportion to her educational opportunities.

The lad entered the University of Königsburg when he was
sixteen years of age and acquitted himself brilliantly in mathematics and philosophy. Following his graduation, he supported
himself for a time by tutoring in private families and lecturing to
military groups on the "art of fortification." In 1755 he was given
the lowly post of private lecturer in his Alma Mater. After fifteen
years without advancement, though he had twice applied for a
professorship, he was unexpectedly awarded the Chair of Logic
and Mathematics. His slowness in achieving merited recognition

may be ascribed to his unimpressive personality. A tiny man, barely five feet in height, and weighing only a little over a hundred pounds, he had a weak voice and a diffident manner. It is said that his chest was concave and his right shoulder deformed, a result, probably, of malnutrition in childhood.

He was never married. For thirty-five years he dined at a table d'hôte, but in 1790 he made a change in his domestic arrangements and began having his meals at home. With this change he initiated a system of guest-dinners which grew into a sort of institution. He arranged with a score of friends for each to dine with him regularly on a certain day of the week. Including himself, he continued to have at least three for dinner (one for each of the graces) and sometimes as many as nine (one for each of the Muses). For his breakfast he had only a few cups of tea. After he had drunk the tea, he allowed himself a pipeful of tobacco. Dinner, his single meal of the day, began punctually at one o'clock and lasted until three o'clock at the earliest and frequently later. There was wine together with a large variety of dishes to which each guest helped himself according to his taste and digestive abilities. It was, however, an intellectual rather than a gastronomic feast.

For his dinner companions Kant preferred young men. As a long-time teacher it seems natural that he should do this, although his former pupil and secretary, Wasianski, who later became his best biographer, suggests that the philosopher chose young men because they were less likely to become seriously ill and so cause him anxiety. If a close friend became sick, Kant manifested the greatest solicitude. If recovery ensued, he rejoiced; if death resulted, he became sternly tranquil. Death he understood as a permanent state that "extinguished the agitations of suspense."

He was fond of long walks unaccompanied by a companion, though his old servant, Lampe, was accustomed to trail along with an umbrella if the weather seemed threatening. Kant's reasons for walking alone were based on considerations of health. If he had a companion, he would talk; if he talked, he would breathe through his mouth; if he breathed through his mouth, he would invite coughs, colds, hoarseness, and pulmonary derangements. As a sensible man, therefore, he walked alone and breathed through his nose.

It was his habit to sit in his study at the twilight of evening and gaze out reflectively on the old tower of Lobenicht as it melted into the gathering darkness. When some poplars in an intervening garden grew so tall as to interfere with the view, the philosopher was quite unable to pursue his accustomed meditations. The cogitative vine had lost its prop-pole. Fortunately, the owner of the garden was an understanding man, and when he learned of Kant's distraction and the cause therefor, he cropped the trees and removed the impediment to rational thinking.

One of Kant's foibles was the meticulous regularity of his habits. He went to bed exactly at ten and arose precisely at five, and up to 1790 he went for a walk at three-thirty, on the minute. To guard against chill he kept his study as nearly as possible to a temperature of seventy-five degrees.

He detested sweat as a sort of watery excrementation. He would not wear garters for fear of impeding the circulation in his legs and was driven to a great extremity, it appears, to find a substitute. The best he could do was to contrive an affair consisting of a watch-spring in a wheel around which was wound an elastic cord divided at each loose end to form a "Y." On either side of the trousers in front was a "watch-pocket" with a small hole in the bottom. The gadget was placed in a pocket and the loose ends of the cord drawn through and down to the stocking where they were attached by hooks. We are told on good authority that the contraption was not an unqualified success.

In keeping with his anxious attention to his health he had a great interest in medical science. He was enthusiastic over a theory advanced by the Scottish physician, Brown—called the "Brunonian theory" after the Latinized name of the originator—which held that all disease was due either to a lack or to an excess of stimulus. He was impressed by Beddoe's essays on the cure of consumption and a method advocated by Reich for the cure of fevers. He did not think well, however, of Jenner's discovery of vaccination against smallpox which, as it turned out, was the only one of the four innovations possessed of any merit. He bore a great prejudice against beer and ascribed all manner of illness to beer-guzzling.

Kant, like many persons whose minds are occupied with abstractions, had a prodigious memory for things of an intellectual nature but a very poor memory for the common affairs of life. When he reached the approximate age of seventy-five, his associates noticed, as the first evidence of memory failure, that he was becoming repetitious in his conversation. Strangely, the philosopher himself also was aware of it and to provide against embarrassment he began preparing each day a syllabus for the next day's conversations. But he lost his programs with such pitiful regularity that the system availed him and his listeners no comfort. As time went on, evidences of intellectual decay became apparent. He developed extravagant theories to explain events not accounted for by known causes. He blamed electricity for an epizootic which was killing the cats of Basle, Copenhagen, and Vienna. The headaches which dulled his memory were ascribed to the same malign force. True, there were times when his mind seemed to function with its pristine clarity, and his friends were encouraged to hope that he might regain his former intellectual vigor. By the time he had reached his seventy-eighth birthday, however, it was obvious that there was no ground for such optimism. He had always had, among his many other lovable traits, great patience and forbearance; but now he was impatient of slight delays, and, indeed, between his petulance and his confused sense of time, he was inclined to complain of delay even when his wishes were served with the greatest celerity.

His memory worked backwards—the more distant an event in his experience, the better he could recall it. In his youth he had been an ardent student of literature, and later, when he could not remember a single incident of yesterday, he could yet recite long passages from the German and Latin classics with perfect precision and fluency. At times he seemed to comprehend his condition for on one occasion, after a minor *faux pas*, he exclaimed apologetically, "Gentlemen, I am old and childish; you must treat me as a child."

He became increasingly unsteady on his legs, and one day early in his seventy-ninth year he fell while walking in the street. Although he suffered no physical injury, he seemed content thereafter to avoid all unnecessary physical exertion. A few months later he was so unsteady that he could scarcely get about his home. While sitting, he was likely to fall forward, especially if he dozed, which he was very likely to do. On one occasion he nodded into some lighted candles which set his night-cap afire, and he suffered minor burns of the hands in removing the *chapeau flamboyant*.

He had frequent delusions, but his mind was usually amenable to reason and could nearly always be persuaded of their falsity. His old house man, Lampe, who had been a soldier in the Prussian Army for many years and who was an obedient though a stupid and unaffectionate servant, suddenly became so indifferent to his duties that Kant was forced to discharge him. This necessity was very disturbing to the master's peace of mind. In behalf of Lampe, there is reason to believe that he, too, was afflicted with a mental disorder. The new servant, Kauffman, was intelligent and devoted. Had he come into the ménage sooner, Kant's last years might have been more serene.

About this time the rapidly aging philosopher began to complain of abdominal pains which defied all attempts at relief. It is probable that this discomfort was due to sclerosis and thickening of the visceral arteries. The next year he complained of unpleasant dreams, often of terrifying vividness, which awakened him in a state of great agitation. He complained, too, that melodies he had heard in his childhood now oftimes resounded painfully in his ears. He had a rope running from his bed to a bell in the room of his servant and almost every night he called frantically for the faithful Kauffman to come to his rescue from imaginary assassins. It was with the greatest difficulty that the old gentleman could be persuaded to keep a light burning in his room throughout the night and have a cot placed in the corner for Kauffman so that the servant could come to his master's aid instantly.

Kant had never been more than a few miles from his native city of Königsburg, but now he began to make plans for a grand tour. His friends decided not to oppose him in his whim and arranged for a carriage to call for the old professor with his luggage and servant. He had no special objective, he said, but he wanted to travel far and fast. After a dozen miles he ordered the driver to turn around and take him back home with all possible speed.

Some years before, Kant had discovered that he was blind in his left eye. How long the blindness had existed, he had no idea. It is most likely that the loss was occasioned by a retinal hemorrhage, especially since it had occurred without pain and the vision in the other eye was unimpaired. Now, however, the right eye began to fail. The opticians did their best, but they could not improve his sight enough to enable him to read.

Several months after he had celebrated his seventy-ninth birthday, he fell to the floor senseless. He was carried to his bed and though he had recovered most of his faculties fifteen hours later, it is said that he was never the same as before. He would sit silently for long periods of time, apparently depressed and only dimly conscious of what was going on about him. No mention of paralysis is made and presumably none occurred but there can be no doubt that he had suffered some degree of cerebral hemorrhage and it was the cause of his collapse. Wasianski, who had tried to enforce a dietary regime of his own conception, blamed the fall on the fact that the old professor had surreptitiously obtained and eaten some bread and English cheese the previous day. Poor Kant had achieved transcendental philosophy only to have transcendental dietetics thrust upon him!

During the years of his decline Kant was occasionally visited by a physician designated as "Doctor A." It appears that a consultation was held by two or three doctors with respect to the abdominal pain which plagued the aged patient and that no diagnosis of the cause was made. Now, however, Doctor A began making frequent visits. He was a kindly man who refused pay for his efforts and who, by his presence rather than by his medicines, was able to contribute a modicum of comfort to a distraught patient.

For several months Kant continued his gradual descent toward the vegetative level. He was practically blind and at times failed to recognize old friends either by voice or by name. But he could repeat a lecture on Kepler's laws of planetary motion or give an accurate account of the customs of the Moors of Barbary. Finally he refused all food and took to his bed, where he lay at first stuporous, then deeply unconscious. On February 4, 1804, he died.

His symptoms have been described in detail because they afford a perfect example of the tragic disintegration of a great and noble intellect under the blight of cerebral arteriosclerosis.

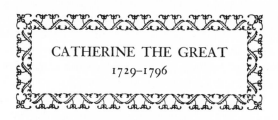

CATHERINE THE GREAT
1729-1796

For centuries the city of Stettin at the mouth of the Oder was a bone of contention among the dogs of war. Finally, in 1720, during the reign of Frederick Wilhelm I, it was ceded to Prussia by the terms of the Peace of Stockholm. The troops with which Frederick garrisoned the place were in charge of General Prince Christian August of Zerbst-Domburg whose Lutheran conscience rejoiced in service to a God and a king with practically identical ideologies.

The General was cousin to the reigning prince of Anhalt-Zerbst who was old and childless. The duty of providing an heir for that principality devolved upon Christian August so he, as a very proper first step, sought and secured a wife.

Johanna Elizabeth, princess of Holstein-Gottorp, was only fifteen years of age at the time of her marriage; Prince Christian August was thirty-seven. Despite her youth, Johanna, who was one of the twelve children of the Bishop of Lubeck, ruled her family from the start. The General was away most of the time, but when at home he was a docile husband and recognized his wife's authority. His marital philosophy was, perhaps, expressed by an inscription sometimes seen above the signature of the proprietor in old-time German taverns—"*Ich bin der Herr in diesem Haus und was meine Weib sagt ist gesetz.*" At any rate it seems that their union was not disturbed by conjugal infelicity. Johanna was of the same religious faith as her husband, but he was apparently more devout than she.

Christian August, like everyone else in the hire of Frederick Wilhelm, was poorly paid, and life in Stettin held much less charm for Johanna than did life in the brilliant court of Brunswick. This circumstance, together with the seeming finality of marriage in one so young, probably aggravated the nervous instability which manifested itself a little later in her life.

Johanna had a first cousin who had married a daughter of Peter the Great and left a son with claims upon the thrones of both Sweden and Russia. Also, she had a brother who was engaged to the youngest daughter of Peter, but smallpox intervened to carry him off before the wedding day arrived. To Johanna nothing else in life was as important as this Russian connection, tenuous and trifling as it seemed to be. She insisted that Christian August should announce their marriage, which was plainly a German affair, to the court of Russia. The husband dutifully composed and sent the unexciting announcement to Empress Catherine I.

After a few months Johanna was obviously pregnant. A son was hoped for and perhaps even expected, but Johanna brought forth a daughter. Although this unhappy choice of nature was a severe blow to Johanna, the General accepted it with true Lutheran resignation. Johanna's immediate post-partum condition was not good. During the preoccupation with the mother, an unnoticed pan of charcoal which had been used to warm the room and the baby set fire to the floor and the lives of both mother and infant were imperiled. The child was named Sophie Auguste Fredrike in honor of three living aunts, and bore the title of Princess Anhalt-Zerbst. In the family circle Sophie was usually called "Fike." About eighteen months after the birth of Sophie, Johanna bore a crippled son. It frequently happens that in the excess of affection which a mother lavishes upon her afflicted child, her other, healthy children are made to suffer neglect. Sophie, in her memoirs as Catherine II, says her mother bore a crippled son "whom she loved idolatrously. I was merely endured and was often harshly and vehemently scolded and not always with justice. I felt all this without being, however, quite clear in my knowledge."

The son, Wilhelm Christian, died at the age of twelve, and

after his death "dissection" revealed a congenitally dislocated hip to have been the source of his disability. A second son came to fill the void left in Johanna's life by the death of Wilhelm. He was named Fritz and apparently was a healthy child, but his neurotic mother insisted that he was sickly and she wasted money, which she could ill afford, sending him first to one health resort and then to another. Eventually two more children, both girls, were born and both perished in infancy. Thus, of five children born to Johanna and Christian August, only two, Sophie and Fritz, were destined to attain adulthood.

As a child, Sophie was plain in appearance. She was sensitive, and though she felt the lack of maternal affection, she was self-contained and obeyed her mother's commands. She was imaginative and, influenced perhaps by her mother's constant chatter about kings and queens, she very early began to entertain visions of the regal life. It is said that at the age of eight she led a playmate to a friendly Catholic priest who amused himself with palmistry and asked the father to presage a crown for her little friend. The monk felt unable to grant her request but, instead, made the prophecy for Sophie herself.

The education of Sophie was placed in the hands of her German tutor, Pastor Wagner, and a French governess known by the familiar name of "Babet." Babet was a clever mademoiselle, endowed with a stable nervous system and shrewd good sense. Her influence upon little Sophie, coming at a time of life when impressions cut deepest and endure longest, must have been tremendous. It is said that Babet frequently read or recited the comedies of Molière to her pupil and that the author's sarcastic treatment of physicians caused Sophie to distrust all doctors for many years thereafter. Sophie always cherished the fondest memories of Babet but invariably denounced Pastor Wagner for a blockhead. The sprightly and slightly cynical mental attitude of the governess was far more attractive for Sophie than the pious gloom and heavy pedagogy of the pastor.

Early in life Sophie became accustomed to the atmosphere of the sick room. Her first brother was a cripple all the twelve years of his life and if her second brother lacked anything to make him a complete emotional wreck, it was supplied by the neurotic and oversolicitious Johanna. At the age of seven, Sophie was stricken by her first serious illness. While kneeling in bedtime prayer, there was a sudden stitch in her side quickly followed by a cough, fever, and delirium. She lay continuously on her left side for a period of three weeks, she recalls, and when she was able to sit up, it was noticed that her body "had taken on the form of a Z." The "right shoulder was higher than the left, the backbone had a zig-zag line, and left shoulder was hollow." Her parents enjoined secrecy on the part of the servants and sought out "a skillful man who knew how to heal dislocations." A strange choice was made; the local executioner was summoned. He prescribed morning massage with the saliva of a girl who had not yet had breakfast, thereby assuring a plentiful supply of the medicament. Then he made a kind of strait jacket—of what material is not disclosed—which was applied and was not to be removed even momentarily except in case of absolute necessity. Apparently he relished the change to constructive effort, for he came every other day to adjust the brace. The patient wore this uncomfortable contraption for more than three years, after which she resumed her status as the one healthy child of the family.

Without doubt little Sophie had a pleurisy and in all probability a pneumonia with it as the basic cause of her illness. It was left-sided and the partial immobilization which she accomplished by lying on the side gave relief from the pain. Since the pleurisy was well defined, it is likely that there was some effusion, that is, empyema which, fortunately, was not virulent enough to claim her life as empyema is wont to do in the absence of surgical drainage. The inflamed pleura set up reflex spasm of the intercostal muscles of the affected side and they combined with pleural adhesions to produce fixation in a posture of deformity. The executioner should probably be credited with a good job. The torso came straight, and in later years Catherine was inclined to ascribe her fine, queenly carriage to the molding effect of the strait jacket applied by a conscientious public servant. About three years after her release from splintage Sophie was given a preview of her destiny.

Elizabeth Petrovna, youngest child of Peter the Great, had seized the throne of Russia from Empress Anna Leopoldovna by means of a military and political coup. The new Empress, who was unmarried, immediately took steps to provide a successor by adopting her nephew, Karl Peter Ulrich, whom she made Grand Duke Peter Feodorovich. The choice was a completely foolish one. The Empress was possessed of a frustrated and distorted maternal instinct and she selected Peter out of purely emotional impulses. The boy was physically weak and subject to frequent attacks of acute illness. Moreover, he was so dim-witted that at the age of seventeen he could scarcely read or write. He was a proper subject for institutional care. The Empress wanted a wife for Peter, and for reasons which can be explained only at length, she settled upon Sophie for what appeared a great honor but was in truth a great martyrdom.

Sophie's father, in his stanch Lutheranism, deprecated the betrothal since it required his daughter to disavow the faith of her people and to embrace in its stead that of the Greek church. But Frederick of Prussia was afraid that if Christian August refused Elizabeth, she might select one of the many daughters of August the Strong, king of Poland, for the wife of the Grand Duke. Such a marriage would ally Poland with Russia, a consummation which Frederick devoutly wished to prevent. The pressure was more than Christian August could withstand. Little Sophie and her mother, who was hysterical with joy at the prospect, made the journey to Moscow and plans for the wedding moved apace. Suddenly Sophie was again stricken with pneumonia. She was extremely sick, but despite the sixteen bleedings which the court physicians performed on her, she managed to survive and to regain her usual good health.

It seemed incomprehensible that illness should strike at this time. The first attack had come eight years before while she was saying her prayers under the benediction of Lutheranism; the next when she was preparing to abandon the Lutheran faith for that of the Greek church. It was not too much to expect consistency from Heaven. This made no sense, but religion must have some use. If it contradicts itself, it might yet do all right as a political instrument. When her illness was at its height and her mother wished to have a Lutheran clergyman called, Sophie executed a masterly stroke—she asked for a Russian priest instead. On June 28, 1744, she was confirmed in the Greek Orthodox church and given the name, Catherine Alexeievna. The marriage followed late in August. The wedding night, says Catherine, was uneventful and every succeeding night for the next nine years was exactly like the first.

The failure of Catherine to become pregnant within the expected time was to Empress Elizabeth a matter of grave concern. Though she must have observed Peter's weakness for dolls and tin soldiers, his disrespectful behavior in church, his delight in abusing and humiliating Catherine in public, his grimaces, and his vulgarities, it seems never to have occurred to her mind that the Grand Duke was a poor, sickly moron without the intellectual or emotional instincts of a normal young man. She charged willful prevention, and Catherine, from a maidenly sense of modesty, made no attempt at self-exoneration. The unnatural position in which Catherine found herself induced a train of nervous symptoms. She began to have frequent severe headaches, her appetite failed, and she was troubled with sleeplessness. At the time of her marriage, she was a plump, rosy-complexioned girl whose good looks lay almost entirely in her healthy appearance. But now she had grown thin and pale, and her face wore a harried expression. Certain intimate friends, who knew where the trouble was, took a realistic view of the situation and met it with practical measures. A young chamberlain of the Grand Duke, a Sergei Saltikov, was glad to come to the aid of a young woman in distress of that particular sort. In December, 1752, Catherine had a miscarriage. In the following July the misfortune again befell her. On the twentieth of September the next year she bore a living son. The delight of Empress Elizabeth knew no bounds. She named the child Paul and virtually kidnapped him when she had him taken to her private apartments where she arranged a nursery and devoted herself wholeheartedly to his care.

Paul turned out to be an ugly weakling. In fact, he resembled Peter so closely that the resemblance is often cited as evidence that he was Peter's child. But Sergei Saltikov, the putative father, had a brother Peter whom Catherine describes as "a fool in the fullest sense of the word and who had the stupidest physiognomy I have ever seen in my life—great leaden eyes, a turned up nose, and a mouth always half open." So either way, Paul's paternity had a catch in it.

Apparently Grand Duke Peter did not deny fathering his wife's son, but "after my confinement," says Catherine, "he usually slept in his own chambers." He seemed to feel a kind of uneasiness over his inexplicable parenthood but was able to submerge it in occupation with his toy soldiers.

Catherine's miscarriages were ascribed to indiscretions. In the first instance she is alleged to have ridden horseback on a short but hasty journey a day or two before symptoms of impending miscarriage appeared. In the second, she was said to have been caught in a storm while duck hunting and to have lain wet and chilled in a leaky tent all the night before the premature birth occurred. Such explanations must, of course, be accepted with a certain amount of reservation. Miscarriages are the spoor of syphilis and lacking the arbitraments of the laboratory we must have suspicions. Apart from Paul, who is regarded as a lunatic and whose reign was an invitation to patriotic murder, little is known of Catherine's children. Paul was certainly of a constitutionally inferior type, but if he bore any of the tell-tale stigmata of congenital syphilis they have not been described. It is well known, of course, that Peter the Great was syphilitic, but Catherine and Paul were not of his blood. Sergei Saltikov was a gay blade, however, and could very well have had any or all of the venereal diseases. In all Catherine had five living children. After Paul came the Grand Duchess Anna who died in infancy. The cause of her death is unknown. Her father was Count Poniatovsky. In 1762 a boy, Bobrinsky, was born, and subsequently there were two girls, all credited to lover Gregory Orlov.

On Christmas Day, 1761, Empress Elizabeth Petrovna died at the age of fifty-two and the moronic Grand Duke became Peter III. His reign covered a period of but six months. To his infantile mind his empire was simply another toy. It was fun to pull a string here and see who jumped there. His silly ukases and absurd behavior threatened the integrity of the nation. He was so stubborn in his idiocies that Catherine could see no way out but to depose him and seize the throne in her own name. The stratagem devised to this end was quickly and successfully executed. The Grand Duke blustered, then surrendered abjectly, and was placed under guard. Catherine's accession followed automatically. After about a week, Peter's guards, tiring of their work, killed their prisoner and freed themselves. The actual murder was probably committed by Alexei Orlov, brother of Catherine's lover, Gregory Orlov. Alexei was reported to have given Peter a drink of poisoned vodka and then to have stifled his screams by strangulation. Although it is not recorded that Catherine punished Alexei or other members of the guard, it is generally believed that she neither wished nor intended to have Peter destroyed.

Following her accession, the remarkable genius of Catherine shone forth in its greatest brilliance. She possessed a masculine intellect, a strong will, admirable judgment, and great political tact. She applied all her energy and talent to the betterment of the lot of the Russian people and to the expansion and consolidation of the Russian Empire.

Catherine's health, on the whole, was excellent. She ate and slept little, consumed great quantities of snuff and strong coffee, and worked twelve to fifteen hours daily. For many years she had a Dr. Rogerson for physician to herself and her court. Rogerson was a Scot who concerned himself with the care of his patients and nothing else, and the Empress was very fond of him. She had a great fear of venereal disease, and her lovers were subjected to examination by Rogerson, sometimes for safety, it seems, and sometimes for purposes of discipline. She knew the prophylactic value of humiliation.

Catherine built a hospital for the care of the venereally infected. It could accommodate about fifty patients. She also endowed a foundling hospital to discourage abortion and infanticide. A citizen named Smolin wrote her a letter rebuking her for building an institution which could only serve to encourage immorality, asserting that more and more illegitimate children would be born. It would seem that Citizen Smolin credited concupiscence with more forethought than it is commonly believed to possess.

In the year 1771 a fearful epidemic of smallpox broke out in Moscow. Local authorities were helpless in the face of the resulting panic. Catherine sent to England for a physician named Dimsdale who was advocating the control of smallpox by inoculation. Dimsdale was elderly, financially comfortable, and loath to leave his native country, but he finally persuaded himself that it was his duty to go. Catherine was among the first to take advantage of the new method of immunization. Most of the nobles and members of the court who had never had the disease followed the example bravely set by their empress. A number of hospitals were opened for the many victims, but the populace, who had got the idea that the doctors had brought the epidemic to Moscow, would have nothing to do with either doctors or hospitals. Instead they put their faith in the Virgin at the Vavarsky Gate. Hundreds of victims in all stages of the disease were massed at the feet of the wonder-working virgin, where they lay day and night polluting the entire neighborhood. The doctors were in despair. The Bishop of Moscow, Father Ambrosius, thought to assist by having the Virgin carried away under cover of darkness. But when he appeared before his people and ordered them to take their stricken relatives back to their homes, they became a howling mob. The priest fled before their anger but was caught and torn to pieces. At this juncture Catherine summoned a regiment of troops and placing her lover, Gregory Orlov, in command, called for the restoration of order. Orlov was considered a no-account gigolo, but fortified by a sense of immunity against the contagion, and galvanized by his mistress' show of confidence in him, he quickly forced the public into compliance with measures recommended by the physicians. The epidemic was checked forthwith. This historic instance of the suppression of an epidemic by police regulation is probably the precedent from which has issued our modern public health departments with their vested authority to impose any measures necessary for protection of the health of the citizens.

Catherine had, all told, one husband and twelve lovers. It is generally believed that she was a nymphomaniac. Her sexual passion seemed to advance with her years so that eventually she became that most repulsive of all female creatures—an aged nymphomaniac. She has her defenders who urge that she was affectionate rather than licentious, but strong presumptive evidence indicates that the reverse was true. She should, however, be given whatever consideration is due for practicing a restrained promiscuousness; she had only one lover at a time. Moreover, she let neither love nor lust interfere with her determination to govern the Russian people to the best of her great ability. Her most famous lover was Potemkin, a man possessed of considerable literary and military skill. He was dismissed by Catherine for reasons not fully recorded and left soon thereafter for the south of Russia. He died of typhus shortly, and it is said that when she received the news of his death, her imperial majesty fainted three times. Her biographers agree that Empress Catherine was a woman of great personal charm; her lovers assert that she was beautiful beyond compare. It is known that she had a tall and graceful figure, blue eyes, and abundant black hair. When she was amused, her laugh was joyous; when she was angered, her invective was eloquent. She detested growing old and employed all the cosmetic artifices of her day to conceal the ravages of time. Before she was sixty, she had lost all her teeth and that fact was a source of great embarrassment, for satisfactory dentures had not yet been devised.

With the passing of the years, the Empress became very heavy. She had had two miscarriages and borne five children and she spent much time on her feet. These circumstances plus an inherent weakness of the vein walls conspired to produce severe varicosities of the lower extremities. In the last three or four years of her life her legs were so badly swollen that she could stand only with the greatest difficulty and had to be conveyed from room to room by means of a wheel chair. Finding that the court doctors could not arrest the advance of age nor cure her swollen legs, she closed her doors against them and placed herself in the hands of a notorious quack named Lambro Cazzoni who prescribed foot baths of ice-cold sea water. It is said that she seemed to improve a little at first as ailing persons are wont to do after a change of doctors, whether the change is ultimately for better or for worse.

On the morning of November 6, 1796, the Empress arose as usual, had her customary five cups of coffee, and then plunged into the daily routine of work. She saw her lover, Zubov, and her secretaries and sent them to their tasks. She then retired to her dressing room. The attendants in the antechamber awaited her call, but it failed to come. Her private secretary was summoned, knocked at the door, received no answer, then entered the apartment. Catherine was lying on the floor gasping and unconscious. Her physicians were called while attendants struggled to place her limp bulk on a mattress which had been torn from a bed and placed

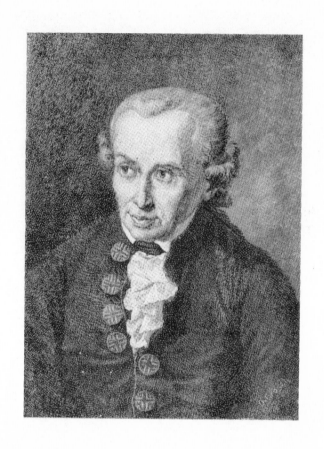

IMMANUEL KANT

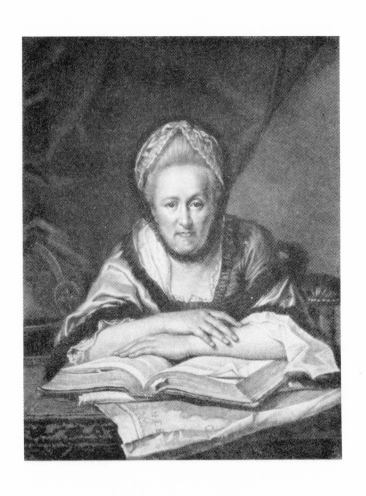

CATHERINE THE GREAT

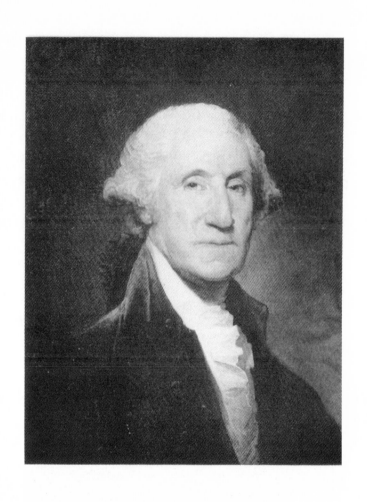

GEORGE WASHINGTON

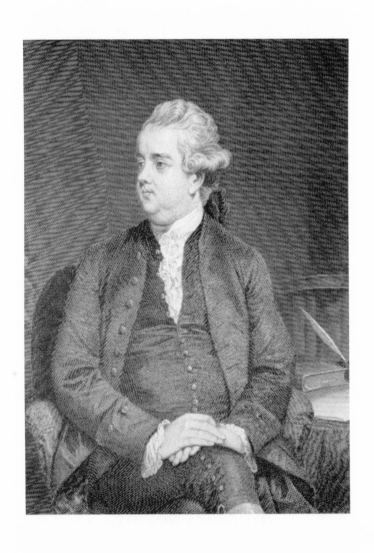

EDWARD GIBBON

on the floor. The doctors arrived, bled her and applied blisters to her feet. The Grand Duke Paul came, looked, said nothing, and departed. The sick woman was restless at first, but after a while she became quieter. Her breathing was deep and regular for the first twenty-four hours, then it was imperceptible one minute and stertorous the next—of a crescendo or Cheyne-Stokes type. In the late evening of the second day she died.

Catherine was unquestionably a victim of high blood pressure associated with arteriosclerosis. Because of cerebral vascular disease, the last years of her life had been marked by a decline in the mental vigor which distinguished the first three decades of her reign. Her death was occasioned by cerebral hemorrhage.

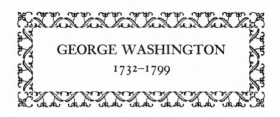

So much has been written of Washington's great physical strength and endurance that it comes as a surprise to most of us when we first learn that in his lifetime the Father of His Country had no less than ten attacks of serious illness and that on at least two occasions his life was despaired of by his physicians. That he survived and was able to accomplish as much as he did is a tribute to both his vitality and his resoluteness of purpose.

Because neither preventive nor curative medicine had yet become a science, it is undoubtedly true that in Washington's time the average citizen suffered from serious infectious disease much more commonly than is the case today. The southernmost of the original thirteen colonies were then so malarious that most of the inhabitants were affected with the disease at one time or another. Because of Washington's strong predilection for life in the open, he undoubtedly had malaria in either an active or a dormant form practically all his life. Some of his bouts of chills and fever were probably seasonal reactivations of the chronic form of the disease; others, most likely, represented newly acquired infections. But apart from his attacks of malaria and the high morbidity resulting from all sorts of diseases among the colonists, it would seem that he suffered more than his just share of sickness.

Little seems to be known of his mother's family, though it is stated that Washington's personal appearance was a heritage from the maternal stock. His paternal grandfather, Lawrence Washington, died at thirty-seven and his father, Augustine Washington, at forty-nine. The latter was twice married. In his will he describes his marriages as "ventures," without intention, it is thought, of appearing either humorous or cynical. George was his fifth child and the first by the second "venture." The mother, Mary Ball Washington, lived to die of cancer of the breast at the age of eighty-one. She had little education and in her later years humiliated her famous son by totally unfounded complaints of poverty and filial neglect.

Perhaps it was the poor family record of longevity as much as his own frequent experience of illness which caused Washington to live, from about the age of thirty, in a state of continuous expectation of death. A haunting sense of mortality is revealed abundantly in letters to friends and relatives, in his diary, and in the doctor's accounts of his illnesses. It did not, however, seem to oppress him greatly, for he always insisted that he was not afraid to die, and his conduct in the presence of danger was composed and deliberate.

Some writers on the subject of Washington's health have maintained that he was prematurely aged. In support of their contention is cited the fact that at the age of fifty-seven he was "using a number of false teeth" and also that in 1783 preparatory to reading an address to officers of his army he said, apologetically, "Gentlemen, you will permit me to put on my spectacles for I have not only grown gray but almost blind in the service of my country."

The remark must not be taken over-seriously. At that time it was not generally known that the normal eye becomes "farsighted" about the age of forty and the aid of glasses is always desirable and frequently necessary. The only middle-aged or elderly people who can read fine script or print readily without glasses are those who were nearsighted the first forty years of their lives. Inasmuch as the General at the age of fifty-seven was still "riding to hounds" and several years after that was able successfully to hunt ducks, geese, and turkeys, we may reasonably conclude that his defects of vision were those normally present in persons of middle age. Nor do poor teeth at any age or gray hair at fifty-one necessarily bespeak a worn-out body.

At full maturity, which was about the age of thirty, Washington was said to have stood six feet, three inches in his stockings and to have weighed in the neighborhood of two hundred pounds. He had wide shoulders and hips, huge hands and forearms, and muscular, but not heavy, thighs and calves. His chest, however, was noticeably flat and his complexion bordered on the sallow. He was a methodical man and his diary and letters give us what is believed to be a fairly complete account of his illnesses and indispositions.

The first recorded sickness occurred at the age of seventeen when he was forced to take to his bed because of exhaustion from ague (malaria) and the high fever which accompanied it. Four years later while sojourning on the island of Barbados, whence he had gone with his half-brother, Lawrence, who was vainly seeking relief from pulmonary tuberculosis, George was stricken with smallpox. He notes that he was "strongly attacked" and was bedfast for three weeks. When he emerged from his six weeks' isolation, his face was badly and permanently pitted.

A few weeks after his return from Barbados he suffered "a violent attack of pleurisy which reduced me very low." It has been suggested with good reason that this was tuberculous pleuritis, a likely result of his close association with the consumptive brother who shortly died of his malady. At any rate, George was in poor health for at least two years thereafter. In 1755, at the age of twenty-four, while still weak from an attack of ague, he ventured to accompany the English general, Braddock, on his ill-fated campaign against the French at Fort Duquesne. The expedition had not progressed far before Washington was stricken with what is now commonly called "flu." His diary describes the experience in these words: "Immediately upon leaving the camp at George's Creek on the fourteenth, I was seized with violent fevers and pains in my head which continued without intermission until the 23d following when I was relieved by General Braddock's absolutely ordering the physicians to give me Dr. James' Powders,[1] one of

[1] A nostrum which consisted of a mixture of antimony oxide and calcium phosphate. In full doses it usually produced nausea, sweating, and catharsis, but an emetic action frequently precluded other effects. Antimony, the more potent ingredient, was once widely employed in medicine, but its

the most excellent medicines in the world for it gave me immediate ease and removed my fevers and other complaints in four days time. My illness was too violent to suffer me to ride, therefore I was indebted to a covered wagon for some part of my transportation but even in this I could not continue for the jolting was so great. I was left upon the road with a guard and necessaries to wait the arrival of Col. Dunbar's detachment which was two days' march behind us, the General giving me his word of honor that I should be brought up before he reached the French fort."

After returning to Mount Vernon from the campaign with Braddock, Washington was still in poor health, for he wrote to one of his half-brothers, "I am not able were I ever so willing, to meet you in town for I assure you that it is with some difficulty and much fatigue that I visit my plantations in the Neck; so much has a sickness of 5 weeks duration reduced me." Two years later, in the autumn of 1757, he suffered a violent attack of fever and diarrhoea. He was forced to leave his command of colonial troops and return to Mount Vernon to recuperate. Recovery was slow and tedious. Dr. Craik, his close personal friend as well as physician, warned him that his life was in danger. After four months he was still weak and miserable with frequent attacks of high fever and diarrhoea. Apparently he was suffering from some sort of intestinal infection, the exact nature of which can never be known. The persistence of the malady is indicated in a letter he wrote to a friend: "I have never been able to return to my command since I wrote you last, my disorder at times returning obstinately upon me in spite of the efforts of all the sons of Aesculapius whom I have hitherto consulted. At times I have been reduced to a great extremity and now have too much reason to apprehend my approaching decay [consumption], being visited with several symptoms of the disease. I am now under a strict regimen and shall set out to-

use is now restricted almost entirely to the treatment of certain tropical diseases of protozoan origin. The name derives from an experiment by Paracelsus, in the sixteenth century, who gave the drug as a tonic to a number of monks who were emaciated by fasting. The monks all died, which fact led the experimenter to the conclusion that it was bad medicine for monks. He therefore called it antimony, which means "antagonistic to monks." The chemical name is stibium.

morrow for Williamsburg to receive the advice of the best physician there. My constitution is certainly greatly impaired and nothing can retrieve it but the greatest care and the most circumspect conduct."

It was while on his way to see the Williamsburg specialist that he first met Martha Custis. What the doctor said is not recorded, but we may surmise that the rich little widow did fully as much as the M.D. to dispel the "apprehensions of decay." At any rate the patient recovered his weight and strength rapidly and after a two year courtship rescued Martha from her state of widowhood.

In 1761, Washington was stricken again. He believed that he had malaria, although it may really have been typhoid fever. At the onset he journeyed to Warm Springs but, as he felt himself growing rapidly worse, cut short his stay and hurried home, where he lay bedfast for several weeks. Concerning this illness he wrote: "I was very near my last gasp. My indisposition increased upon me and I fell into a very low and dangerous state." He had barely regained his strength and resumed normal activity when he began again to have chills and fever. This could hardly have been a typhoid relapse; more likely it was another attack of malaria. Recovered from this illness, he enjoyed a six-year period of freedom from any sort of disabling sickness. Then came another round of malaria, followed by a stretch of robust health unequaled in his experience up to this time.

It seems providential that he was never seriously disabled by sickness or accident during the Revolution, when his continuous presence in the field was so vital to its success. It was not until 1786, after the conclusion of the war and his election to the Presidency (but before he had assumed office) that he was again seized with malaria and confined "with ague and fever." This time Dr. Craik "applied the bark" with excellent results. It seems strange that, though the bark of the quinine or cinchona tree had been used against malaria in South America and southern Europe for nearly 150 years, it was not widely employed in North America until about 1800. It was administered in the form of powder, decoction, or extract and was a veritable godsend to the wretched pioneers of the Southeastern states.

Shortly after his assumption of the Presidency, Washington

developed what his doctors called a "malignant carbuncle," or anthrax, which indeed it may have been, though the location of the lesion on the anterior surface of the thigh and its slow evolution are more characteristic of the ordinary staphylococcic type of carbuncle. He was desperately sick and septic, and there can be no doubt but that he missed death by a narrow margin. During this illness he was cared for by Dr. Baird, an eminent New York physician, who attended the patient constantly for many days and nights. That the President believed the illness was destined to have a fatal outcome is evidenced by his admonition to Dr. Baird: "Do not flatter me with vain hopes. I am not afraid to die and therefore can hear the worst." At this time Senator William Maclay reported to a friend: "Called to see the President and every eye full of tears. His life despaired of, his danger imminent and everyone expected that the event of his disorder would be unfortunate."

During his convalescence from the infection Washington wrote: "I have the pleasure to inform you that my health is restored, but a feebleness still hangs upon me and I am much incommoded by the incision which was made in a very large and painful tumor on the protuberance of my thigh. However, the physicians assure me that it has had a very happy effect in removing my fever and will tend very much to the establishment of my general health; it is in a fair way of healing and time and patience only are wanting to remove the evil. I am able to take exercise in my coach by having it so contrived as to extend myself the full length of it."

In 1789, while on a tour of New England, Washington, due, according to Sullivan, "to some mismanagement" in the reception ceremonials at Cambridge, was detained a long time and the weather being inclement, took cold. For several days afterward a severe influenza prevailed at Boston and its vicinity, and was called the "Washington Influenza." The designation has the ring of loyalist slander. Of this attack of illness he wrote, "Myself much disordered by a cold and inflammation in the left eye." There is some evidence that actually he had pneumonia at this time. A year later he wrote: "Within the last twelve months I have undergone more and severer sickness than thirty preceding years afflicted me with. Put it all together I have abundant reason, however, to be thankful I am so well recovered, though I still feel the remains of the violent affection of my lungs; the cough, pain in my breast, and shortness in breathing not having entirely left me."

In 1794, while at Mount Vernon, he hurt his back by "an exertion to save myself and horse from falling among the rocks at the Lower Fall of the Potomac (whither I went on Sunday morning to see the canal and locks)." The injury confined him for some time before he was able again to "ride with ease and safety."

In 1798, after he had finished his second term as president, he "was seized with a fever, of which I took little notice until I was obliged to call for the aid of medicine; and with difficulty a remission thereof was so far effected as to dose me all night on thursday with Bark—which having stopped it, and only weakness remaining, will soon wear off as my appetite is returning." To a correspondent he apologized for not replying sooner, pleading "debilitated health, occasioned by the fever wch. deprived me of 20 lbs of the weight I had when you and I were at Troy Mills Scales, and rendered writing irksome." At this time Washington was wearing false teeth, of which he had two sets made of ivory. Because the ivory was obtained from the mouths of hippopotami, the dentures, with a fine disregard of etymology, were called "sea-horse" teeth. His hearing was bad, as we might expect it to be in one of his age who had suffered so much from respiratory infections. In 1792, so it is said, he remarked to Thomas Jefferson that he was "sensible, too, of a decay of his hearing, perhaps his other faculties might fall off and he not be sensible of it."

The last year of the century was likewise the last year of life for George Washington. Colonel Tobias Lear, his capable secretary and devoted friend, has left a moving account of the final illness. Supplementing Colonel Lear's description of the General's last hours is a joint statement issued by the attending physicians and published in the *Times* of Alexandria the day following demise. The circumstances as gathered from these two sources are as follows:

December 12, 1799, was a day of rain, sleet, snow, and chilling wind at Mount Vernon. Despite the inclemency of the weather, the General, who seemed in excellent health, followed his daily habit of riding about the farm from ten A.M. to three P.M. When he came in, it was noted that the clothing about his neck was wet and ice and snow were clinging to his hair. As dinner was waiting for him, he sat down to eat without changing his clothes. The next morning he complained of a sore throat. He stayed indoors until early afternoon. Then he went out to mark some trees to be cut down. When he returned to the house, he was hoarse, but made light of the condition and insisted on reading aloud to the family. Near bedtime when Colonel Lear suggested that he should take something for the condition, the General replied, "You know I never take anything for a cold; let it go as it came!"

At three o'clock the next morning, Washington called his wife, saying that he thought he was having an attack of ague. He could hardly speak and was breathing with difficulty. Mrs. Washington wanted to get up and fetch a concoction, but her husband forbade her lest she catch cold. At daylight an attempt was made to administer a mixture of molasses, butter, and vinegar, but the patient choked on it and was quite unable to swallow any of it. The overseer of the farm, who had some experience at bleeding, was summoned and commanded to take a pint of blood. This he did, but it gave no relief. Colonel Lear applied "sal volatile" to the throat, rubbing it in gently. The General remarked upon the soreness and pain evoked by the treatment. Next a piece of flannel was moistened with sal volatile and wrapped about the neck while the feet were bathed in hot water. At this juncture Dr. Craik arrived and applied blisters to the throat, withdrew more blood, and attempted to administer a gargle of vinegar and sage tea. He also ordered a brew of vinegar and hot water for vapor inhalation. The patient attempted to use the gargle and came near suffocating. For the third time blood was taken, but the sick man continued to grow worse. Doctors Gustavus R. Brown of Port Tobacco and Elisha Dick of Alexandria arrived and more blood, this time about a quart, was removed. Dr. Dick objected to the bleeding, saying, "He needs all his strength; bleeding will diminish it." But the other two doctors and the General himself overruled the young physician. It was remarked this time that the blood "came slow and thick" (the result of dehydration). Calomel and tartar were offered, and the sick man somehow managed to get some of the medicament down. But it did him no good.

During the afternoon the General insisted upon giving directions concerning his will and sat up in bed for a while. When he lay down again, he was in great distress and extremely restless. About eight P.M. the doctors applied more blisters to the throat and also enveloped his legs and feet in poultices of wheat bran. About ten o'clock he became quieter and, it was thought, breathed a little easier. At eleven-thirty P.M. respiration suddenly stopped.

Doctors Craik and Dick reported that Washington was convinced from the first that his illness would terminate fatally and early in the second day said to them, "I feel myself going. I thank you for your attention but I pray you to take no more trouble for me. Let me go quietly. I cannot last long."

The exact cause of General Washington's death is, among medical men, still a matter of dispute. His physicians first said it was quinsy (peri-tonsillar abscess) and then changed the diagnosis to "cyanche trachealis," an indefinite medical term which was abandoned a half-century later in the surge of more exact medical knowledge. A fairly complete and modern study entitled *The Last Illness and Death of Washington* was made in 1927 by Dr. W. A. Wells of Washington, D. C., who published his findings in the Virginia Medical Monthly for January of that year. It was Dr. Wells' considered judgment that death was caused primarily by an infection, probably streptococcic, with obstruction of the glottis (the aperture between the vocal cords) by inflammatory swelling. In those days nothing whatever was known of bacteriology; consequently the clinical manifestations of the different diseases were not clearly distinguished. As Dr. Wells points out, there is nothing to indicate that the interior of the throat was examined at any time during the fatal illness. Yet the physicians were not negligent. Doctors Craik and Brown had studied in the best medical schools abroad and Dr. Dick, though born and trained in America, had a brilliant mind and the gift of independent thinking. The treatment given, poor as it was, was the best known at the time.

It is to be expected, in view of the scant diagnostic evidence, that there should be a difference of opinion respecting the identity of the ailment which took the life of our first President. Incidental references to the illness as seen in modern medical literature almost invariably call it diphtheria, and that diagnosis appears to be the one generally accepted among physicians. It is quite true that laryngeal diphtheria (membranous croup) typically presents a concatenation of symptoms very much like those described by Washington's doctors and Colonel Lear. In his review of the case, Dr. Wells considers the possibility of diphtheria only to rule it out. He calls attention to the extreme unlikelihood of the disease occurring in a man sixty-seven years of age. Moreover, as he says, from the beginning of his illness, Washington was unable to swallow, a circumstance unusual for diphtheria of the larynx. Too, if the disease were diphtheria, the sick man had to catch it from someone. He had not been away from home for several weeks, and there is no record of sore throat among members of the household or other associates either immediately before or after the fatal illness. It appears probable, therefore, that the streptococcus was the assassin of the man to whom the world is indebted more than to any other for the founding of the United States.

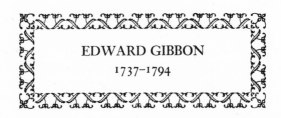

THE FAME of Edward Gibbon derives almost solely from his monumental *History of the Decline and Fall of the Roman Empire*. The professional historian esteems and venerates the six-volume work as a model of diligent research and a masterful presentation of the classical element in Roman history; the layman is impressed and perhaps somewhat dismayed by its sheer bulk.

Gibbon was born at Putney in the county of Surrey, England, the son of Edward Gibbon, Esquire, and Judith Porten Gibbon. His father was moderately wealthy and Edward, Junior, was given the best educational opportunities available in an age of scholars. In his early youth he learned to speak English and French with equal facility, he could write Latin almost as readily as either of the living languages, and eventually he acquired a knowledge of Greek only slightly inferior to his knowledge of Latin. He was the first of six children, "five of whom," he writes, "were snatched away in their infancy."

Despite the high infant-mortality rate of the time due to a multiplicity of causes, the fact that the first-born alone survived the period of infancy immediately suggests the possibility of an Rh-negative mother. Unfortunately the exact ages of the respective infants at death is unknown, but in four of them it appears to have been but a few days or weeks. Gibbon mentions a sister "whose life was somewhat prolonged and whom I remember as an amiable infant." If the mother was truly Rh negative and the daughter happened to be of the same Rh type as the mother, the coincidence would explain the fact of her existence beyond the first few weeks of life.

Gibbon speaks of his own feebleness of constitution and then says: "To preserve and rear so frail a being the most tender assiduity was scarcely sufficient and my mother's attention was somewhat diverted by her frequent pregnancies, by an exclusive passion for her husband and by the dissipation of the world in which his taste and authority obliged her to mingle. But the maternal office was supplied by my aunt, Mrs. Catherine Porten, at whose name I feel a tear of gratitude trickling down my cheek. . . . Many wakeful nights did she sit by my bedside in trembling expectation that each hour would be my last. Of the various and frequent disorders of my childhood my own recollection is dark, nor do I wish to expatiate on so disgusting a topic." He further records that, in a mood of desperation, his family called in every local practitioner from the highest to the lowest in the scale of repute and that his frequent confining illnesses interfered seriously with his early schooling.

Thus he struggled apparently until the age of puberty when the transition from childhood to adolescence brought, as often happens, deliverance from early weaknesses and ailments. In his own words, " . . . as I approached my sixteenth year Nature displayed in my favor her mysterious energies; my constitution was fortified and fixed, and my disorders, instead of growing with my growth and strengthening with my strength, most wonderfully vanished. . . . since that time few persons have been more exempt from real or imaginary ills."

Gibbon was sixteen years of age when his father, scandalized by his son's conversion to Catholicism, took the lad from Oxford and sent him to Lausanne where he was "settled under the roof and tuition" of Mr. Pavilliard, a Calvinist minister. Gibbon declares that at this time he had little proficiency in the arts of fencing and dancing and that some months were wasted in the riding school. "My unfitness to bodily exercise reconciled me to a sedentary life," he says, "and the horse, the favorite of my countrymen, never contributed to the pleasures of my youth." Lord Sheffield

(John Baker Holroyd), author of memoranda on the life and character of Gibbon in addition to a circumstantial account of his final illness, tells of Mr. Pavilliard's confessed astonishment as he gazed on his new pupil, "a thin little figure with a large head disputing and urging with the greatest ability all the best arguments that had ever been used in favor of popery." According to Sheffield, Gibbon later "became very fat and corpulent, but he had uncommonly small bones and was very slightly made."

In May, 1760, two years after his return from Switzerland, Gibbon was pressed into military service when he joined a Hampshire regiment of militia with the rank of captain. During his two and one-half years of army life he was able, apparently, to perform the soldierly requirements of the drill and march without suffering undue physical fatigue, a circumstance which arouses the suspicion that his alleged "unfitness to bodily exercise" was essentially a state of mind. Following his discharge from the militia, he traveled extensively on the Continent before returning to England and the pursuit of a literary career with political punctuations; but it was at Lausanne in June, 1787, that he wrote the last line of the last page of his renowned history. He continued to reside at Lausanne until June, 1793, when he again returned to England in a condition of apparently excellent health. In a letter dated at St. James Street, London, November 11, 1793, however, he wrote Lord Sheffield: "I must at length withdraw the veil before my state of health though the naked truth may alarm you more than a fit of the gout. Have you never observed through my *inexpressibles* a large prominency which, as it was not at all painful and very little troublesome I had strangely neglected for many years? But since my departure from Sheffield Place it has increased (most stupendously) is increasing and ought to be diminished. Yesterday I sent for Farquhar who is allowed to be a very skillful surgeon. After viewing and palpating he desired to call in assistance and has examined it again today with Mr. Cline, a surgeon, as he says, of the first eminence. They both pronounce it a hydrocele (a collection of water) which must be let out by the operation of tapping, but from its magnitude and long neglect they think it a most extraordinary case and wish to have another surgeon, Dr. Baille, present. If the business should go off smoothly I shall be delivered from my burden (it is almost as big as a small child) and walk about in four or five days with a truss. But the medical gentlemen, who never speak quite plain, insinuate to me the possibility of an inflammation, of fever, etc."

Subsequently Gibbon revealed to Sheffield that he had first noticed the swelling thirty-two years before and had at that time consulted Mr. Hawkins, a surgeon, who was unable to decide whether it was due to hydrocele or rupture. As it had occasioned him neither pain nor inconvenience until then, he had done nothing further about it.

A "tapping operation" was performed for the first time about the middle of the month of November and four quarts of a watery fluid were removed, the tumor was diminished to nearly half its former size, and neither inflammation nor fever ensued. With release of fluid-pressure against the secreting surface of the inner scrotal sac, however, a rapid outpouring of exudate resulted, and after a few days the mass was as large as before. Accordingly a second puncture was done a fortnight after the first. But fluid quickly collected again, inflammation was evident, and on January 9, 1794, it was observed that a "considerable degree of fever" was present and the scrotum was ulcerated in several places. The ulcerations probably marked the site of the punctures which the surgeons had made. On January 13 the watery tumor was drained for a third time when "no less than six quarts of fluid" were removed.

On January 14 the patient seemed better, but the next day he complained of pain in the region of the stomach and that evening he was nauseated and suffered much discomfort. About nine o'clock he took a "draught" of opium and went to bed. About ten his pain was not only unrelieved but possibly worse than an hour before. Warm napkins were applied to the abdomen, but the pain persisted until about four o'clock next morning when the sick man said he was feeling much better. At eight-thirty he arose from his bed and declared that he was "*plus adroit*" than he had been for three months past. Shortly he returned to bed unassisted. When, presently, he desired to rise again, his servant persuaded him to remain abed until the surgeon, Mr. Farquhar, who was due at eleven o'clock, should come. When Farquhar arrived at the appointed hour, he found his patient in a state of collapse, but what the surgeon did or attempted to do is not recorded. Presumably he came, saw, and retreated, for it is noted that the servant returned at half past eleven after "attending Mr. Farquhar out of the room." At twelve Gibbon swallowed some brandy and water. He then lay tranquil but seemingly conscious until about 12:45 when it was observed that he had ceased to breathe.

In his report of the *Last Illness and Death of Gibbon*, Lord Sheffield insists, apparently because of the fatal issue, that his friend certainly had a rupture as the basic cause of his trouble. Sheffield was neither a surgeon nor an anatomist, and his assumption that the presence of a hernia was necessary to explain the fatal turn of Gibbon's illness is unwarranted. A closed hydrocele, the sort which tormented Gibbon, has no open connection with the abdominal cavity. True, it may be associated with hernia, but in such case the hernia lies in its own sac or compartment above the hydrocele, each existing independently of the other. Undoubtedly the surgeons introduced infection into the enormously distended sac in the course of their tapping operations, inflammation followed, and death resulted from sepsis. There may have been some extension of inflammation to the abdominal wall contiguous to the upper extremity of the virulently infected sac, but the abdominal discomfort as described was essentially of the referred type due to inflammatory involvement of the testicle and spermatic cord. It was not the type characteristic of acute, spreading peritonitis. It should perhaps be mentioned that the serous exudate commonly found in hydroceles is an excellent culture medium for a large variety of bacteria.

Treatment of hydrocele by puncture-drainage is at best a palliative procedure, almost never curing the condition. Before the advent of surgical cleanliness and appreciation of the value of continuous free drainage for infected cavities, the operation of tapping a hydrocele was fraught with the gravest danger. The "medical gentlemen" who "insinuated the possibility of an inflammation, or fever, etc." in the case of Gibbon were well aware of the hazard involved, but, in view of the great size of the swelling, decided that the patient must accept the risk. Had they but known to make a simple incision two or three inches in length, passing through the walls of the scrotum to permit continuous free drainage as long as it would, they could have saved the life of their illustrious patient.

Under present-day surgery, resection of the inner sac of a hydrocele readily cures the condition. The risk is practically nil and there is no reason for permitting the condition to go on as Gibbon did. Surgery being what it was in his time, however, he probably lived longer as a result of his procrastination.

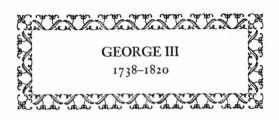

GEORGE III
1738–1820

I<small>N GENERAL</small> the appellation George III falls harshly upon American ears. Most of us have been taught that the third Hanoverian king and the first of the dynasty to be born in England was the author and instigator of oppressive measures which drove the American colonies into revolt against the mother country. Remarkably, a great many Englishmen, who obviously have much more reason than we to regret the Revolutionary War, seem to agree with our teachers.

George was the eldest son of Frederick Louis, prince of Wales, and Princess Augusta of Saxe-Gotha. Both parents were of practically pure German blood. Frederick Louis was a selfish, rebellious, completely erratic person who quarreled with his family, his associates, and his father's ministers. He was probably slightly insane when, to the great relief of everyone, death ended his ridiculous career while his father, George II, was yet upon the throne. Augusta was an energetic and devoted mother, but she was ignorant, stubborn, and obsessed by absolutist ideas. Her daily exhortation to the heir apparent was, "George, when you get to be king, *be* king!"

In his youth George was vain, obstinate, lazy, and inclined to sulk. In his early maturity he was a good physical specimen, above six feet in height, well proportioned and healthy. When he ascended the throne, in 1760, he threw off his lethargy and began a vigorous pursuit of the ideal implanted in his mind by his mother;

he determined to *be* king at once and with a vengeance. With the assistance of an old family friend, the Earl of Bute, a Scotsman who probably didn't like Englishmen anyway, the King managed to oust the Whigs from offices of importance and force the resignation of "the great commoner," William Pitt, first Earl of Chatham. But the English people were not in the mood for absolute monarchy, the King's ministers and advisers proved themselves incompetent, and finally, with the American colonies virtually lost and almost all of Europe aligned against England, George had to admit failure of his autocratic policies. Apparently, however, there was no self-censure in his admission, though it is asserted that in the bitterness of his disappointment he contemplated abdication of his throne.

George was married to Charlotte of Mecklenberg in 1761. His deportment both as husband and father accorded perfectly with the national ideal and won him about all the respect he was ever able to achieve. He is, however, entitled to whatever credit accrues for a certain small contribution to the English vernacular; he is said to have been the first of his nation to use the double interrogative, "What? What?" at the ends of his sentences.

It is now generally known that King George suffered several attacks of mental derangement. One of the most disconcerting of these occurred in the summer of 1788 when, according to McCarthy, his Majesty "was wholly deprived of reason and placed under restraint. . . . According to established law, parliament, without being opened by the Crown, had no authority to proceed to any business whatever." Mr. Fox maintained that the Prince of Wales had "as clear a right to exercise the power of sovereignty as if the king were actually dead." The discussion of the situation was so prolonged that George recovered his faculties before the Regency Bill, framed by the younger Pitt, could be passed.

Modern authorities on mental disease agree that the King was a victim of manic depressive psychosis, which is an essentially benign affective type of psychosis characterized by periods of emotional instability and striking mood swings. There are several subtypes of the disorder which need not be described here. It is doubtful if the victim of manic depressive attacks is ever quite normal minded at any time in his life.

The story of King George's insanity has been well told by Walter R. Bett in a letter published in the British Medical Journal a dozen years ago. The letter reads:

"George III, the bicentenary of whose birth occurred this year, though intelligent, energetic, and a model of domestic propriety, from childhood displayed a mulish obstinacy. This led him consistently to oppose the tremendous intellectual changes which his long and singularly purposeless reign witnessed, and also directly precipitated the American Revolution. His grandfather, George II, had been subject to fits of depression which could be solaced only by music, and his father, Frederick Louis, Prince of Wales, played a pitiful role in English history. On his mother's side there was feeble mindedness verging on insanity.

"The king was twenty-seven years of age when he suffered his first attack of mental aberration in the spring of 1765. It was evidently of short duration and, as it was carefully concealed by the family, the records are incomplete and obscure. One hundred and fifty years ago, on October 24, 1788, he had his second attack which has been intimately described by several witnesses. At a levee the king was noticed to act strangely and to talk incessantly until he became hoarse. He was irritable, petulant, and despotic and soon showed undeniable signs of insanity, delusional in nature, with exacerbations of mania followed by intervals of utter depression. Naturally the Monarch's illness amounted to a political crisis and upon his physicians fell a serious, almost unprecedented, responsibility. Of these the most interesting was Francis Willis (1718–1807) who was then seventy years old.

"Willis had taken holy orders in 1740 and soon afterward was appointed vicar of St. John's, Wapping, and later of Greatford in Lincolnshire. In his spare time he prescribed for his poor parishioners and kept a successful and prosperous lunatic asylum. His medical activities angered the physicians of the neighborhood and, to protect himself, Willis obtained the degree of M.D. from Oxford University in 1759. A man of fine presence, outspoken and cheerful, he possessed an uncanny instinct for knowing what treatment each individual case required. When he was first introduced at Court the King expressed surprise at a clergyman practicing medicine and Willis' protest that the Savior Himself went about healing the sick received the crushing reply, 'Yes, but He had not seven hundred pounds a year for it.' The clerical physician was popular neither with his colleagues nor with his royal patient. George seemed to have disliked him so thoroughly that he could never afterwards hear his name without a shudder. When he became maniacal, Willis did not hesitate to have him confined in a straight-jacket. Some of his treatment was bizarre and open to censure. He allowed the patient to read King Lear which he professed he had never read himself, and he entrusted him with a razor. Of all the Court physicians, Willis was the most sanguine about the King's recovery. Between him and his colleagues feeling at one time became dangerously bitter, especially when a notice was displayed in the ante-room that no one was to see the Monarch without the permission of Francis Willis and his son, John.

"George had altogether five attacks of insanity, the final one in 1810 being precipitated by the illness of his favorite daughter, the Princess Amelia. Contrary to the prognosis of his physicians he did not recover, becoming blind and permanently deranged. While he retained his physical strength almost to the end what he felt most grievously was the waning of his royal prestige. During the 1801 attack Francis Willis was too old to be active himself but he succeeded again in assuming absolute ascendancy over the King through his sons. In 1804, however, the King had seen enough of the Willis family and he was now attended by Samuel Foart Simmons of St. Luke's Hospital who for the first time dispensed correct and judicious treatment. By a strange irony of fate he who was so tragically pursued by the specter of insanity was also pursued at least three times by insane people, including a housemaid who fancied she had a right to the throne, a soldier, and a lieutenant. Unwittingly George III may be said to have helped revolutionize the treatment of the insane in this country after Pinel and the Tukes had paved the way."

According to Overholser, the 1788 attack lasted for five months. It was during this attack, while the King was confined in the Willis asylum, that he informed the Lord Chancellor that he had been knocked down and in other ways subjected to mistreatment. Indignation was widespread and did much to arouse a public demand for more humane treatment of the mentally ill in England.

George died in 1820, and the Prince of Wales, who had been made regent in 1811, ascended the throne as George IV. McCarthy has described in graphic language the last years of the afflicted King: "Stone blind and stone deaf and, except for rare lucid intervals, wholly out of his senses, the poor old King wandered from room to room of his palace, a touching picture with his long, white flowing beard, now repeating to himself the awful words of Milton, 'dark, dark, amid the blaze of noon—irrecoverably dark,' now, in a happier mood, announcing himself to be in the companionship of angels."

The immediate cause of the aged Monarch's death is unknown.

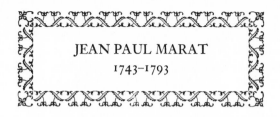

ONE OF THE MOST RABID and ruthless leaders of the French Revolution was Jean Paul Marat who, it happened, was not a Frenchman at all but was born in the town of Boudry in the canton of Neuchâtel, Northwest Switzerland. His father was a Sardinian and his mother was a native of Geneva. Marat is perhaps better known for the manner of his death than for the part he played in the Revolution. Of greater medical interest, however, is the chronic skin disease which, during the last months of his life, nearly drove him insane with an intolerable itching. It is quite possible that by its aggravation of his native cynicism the affliction became a proximate cause of the cruelties which marred his conduct in the Revolution, and it is a matter of history that it made possible his own entrapment and violent death.

A review of his career reveals clearly that Marat's espousal of the Revolution came by his own free choice and not by the resistless dictates of circumstance. His life as moulder of his own future began in 1759 when, following the death of his mother, he left his home and crossed the frontier of France. After a season of futile wandering about the country, he traveled to Bordeaux, where he remained for two years in the study of medicine. There, it is said, he applied his newly found medical knowledge to cure himself of a chronic disease of the eyes. Maintaining an active interest in medicine, he visited Paris, sojourned for a few months in Holland, and then crossed over to London, where after a few years he became a well-known and successful practitioner of his profession. A man of furious energy, he found time despite his large practice to publish a number of articles on philosophical and scientific subjects. The favorable reception given these publications undoubtedly helped their author to obtain the degree of Doctor of Medicine which was conferred at St. Andrews, Edinburgh, in 1775. About this time, issuance of the third volume of Marat's *Philosophical Essays on Man* roused the antagonism of Voltaire, whose imprudent notice of the young essayist redounded to the further benefit of the latter.

In 1777 the Comte d'Artois, afterwards Charles X of France, made Marat physician to his guards with an annual income of two thousand livres and perquisites. Thus established, the young physician quickly acquired an aristocratic clientele and apparently had excellent material and social reasons to be content with his lot. In 1786, however, he resigned his court appointment and retired from the practice of medicine to publish a new translation of *Newton's Optics* in addition to his own *Academic Memoirs or New Discoveries Concerning Light* (*Mémoirs Academiques ou Nouvelle Decouvertes sur la Lumière*).

It is possible that his contact with the aristocratic element in French society infused into his mind a deep hostility against this class. At any rate by the year 1789 he was known as a passionate radical and the editor of *L'Ami du Peuple*, an infamous sheet whose denunciations of the popular party and of select individuals, regardless of party affiliation, brought the editor a short term in prison. But his paranoid brain was aflame with the fire of revolution and nothing short of his own physical destruction could stop him. After making a demagogic attack on the beloved Lafayette, he found it expedient to flee to London to avoid arrest. However, taking advantage of the confusion which existed everywhere in France, he soon dared to return to Paris and resume, in secret, the publication of *L'Ami du Peuple*. Probably as a result of his constant hiding in cellars, sewers, and all sorts of foul, damp places when the tides of his changing fortune were at low ebb, he developed a skin disease accompanied by a terrific pruritis, an affliction which persisted despite his return to a more nearly normal manner of living.

To gain respite from the unbearable itching, he was accustomed to spend many hours daily in a warm bath, where, with his body immersed to the level of the lower ribs and with paper and pen on a stool before him he wrote impassioned editorials for his *L'Ami du Peuple*. He was thus engaged on the evening of July 13, 1793, when he overheard a feminine voice begging the guard for admittance in order that she might communicate important information concerning a Girondist plot which was about to be hatched in Caen against the Mountainists. The unsuspecting Marat called to the guard to let the visitor in, which was done. She was an attractive young woman who identified herself as a fellow partisan by the name of Charlotte Corday and she presented a roster bearing names of the alleged conspirators. Marat read the list and then exclaimed angrily, "They shall soon be guillotined!" At this juncture the girl quickly drew a knife from the folds of her dress and drove the blade full length into the left side of Marat's chest. The astonished victim cried out, "*À moi! Mon ami*," and expired immediately.

The weapon was found to be an ordinary dinner knife which had been ground to a sharp point. Charlotte insisted that in killing Marat she was actuated by purely patriotic considerations, but it has been stated on good authority that the true reason was a mad desire to avenge the death of her lover who had been slain by direction of the "Assassination Committee" of the Mountainist party. Examination of Marat's body disclosed that the blade had entered the chest between the ribs and, passing completely through the lung, had gashed the aorta. Death resulted from internal hemorrhage.

The nature of Marat's skin ailment was discussed in the *Journal of the American Medical Association* of September 2, 1933, in response to a query made by this writer. Says the *Journal*: "In the fourth edition of his Marat inconnu, Doctor Augustin Cabanes has dedicated a chapter to Marat's ailments. He quotes Souberbielle, who was both the friend and the physician of the famous demagogue, to the effect that he suffered atrociously during his last five months from a *dartre* which began about the scrotum and perineum, from which it spread over almost the entire body. It was accompanied by such severe pruritis that Marat was compelled toward the end to pass most of the time in the bath tub where Charlotte Corday ended his career. The *dartre* of the older French dermatologists corresponds to what is now termed Pityriasis Simplex, which many consider to be of microbic origin. Marat had suffered severely from neurasthenia as far back as 1774, almost twenty years before his death. The privations which he endured in later years plus overwork and excessive indulgence in coffee all contributed to the prominence of his cutaneous symptoms."

The term *Pityriasis Simplex* designates a disorder of the sebaceous glands of the skin which in its most elementary form is represented by ordinary dandruff (*Seborrheoa Sicca*). It commonly occurs on the scalp, beard, and pubic regions. In the last-named situation, according to Ormsby, "the itching is often more severe than occurs when the disease is limited to the scalp." On any of these surfaces the condition may shade insensibly into those described under *Dermatitis Seborrheica*. Tobias also states that "*Dermatitis Seborrheica* may result from *Pityriasis Simplex* as a result of irritation and infection with staphylococcus alba." Perhaps the type of irritation best calculated to convert *Pityriasis Simplex* into *Dermatitis Seborrheica* in its most aggravated form is scratching, and we may be sure that the neurotic Marat indulged freely in that fatal luxury. The effect was not only a tremendous intensification of the severity of the dermatitis, but also a gradual extension of the inflammatory process from the genital region to large areas of skin adjacent to the original focus. It was indeed a terrible affliction. Even today a case of the sort is not easily cured though the suffering of the patient may be largely mitigated.

In view of the extremity to which his ailment had reduced Marat, one is forced to wonder to what end Marat would have come had he escaped the hand of the assassin.

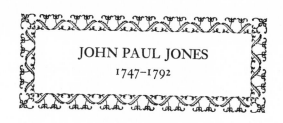

IN ALL THE HISTORY of naval achievement, few men indeed have done so much with so little as did the American Revolutionary hero, John Paul Jones. Regrettably, it was not merely a dearth of ships, men, and material that hampered the genius of the valiant commander. Official incompetence and jealousy aided and abetted by private rascality also played a part in frustrating his zealous efforts to muster an effective fighting squadron against the British navy. But despite the overwhelming odds against him, he was yet able to strike blows that rattled the teeth and addled the brains of the lords of the British Admiralty.

Born John Paul, he was the son of a Scottish gardener who lived in the village of Arbigland on the north shore of Solway Firth. Precisely why he assumed the surname "Jones" is not known. It seems very likely, however, that the change was made to conceal his identity. The circumstances are these: In May, 1770, aboard a trader at the West Indian port of Tobago, Paul exercised his legal right as captain of a vessel to sentence one of the crew to a flogging for what in those days was considered good and sufficient reason. The offender, Mungo Maxwell, who was a Scot and fellow townsman of Paul, took his punishment in poor spirit and immediately thereafter lodged a complaint against the Captain in the Court of Vice Admiralty. Paul, barely able to get about with acute malaria, was summoned to give an account of the affair. The surrogate questioned the Captain and inspected the bared back of the complainant. The marks of the lash were plainly visible, but the damage was obviously trivial and the charge was dismissed. After the hearing Maxwell loafed around the water front for a month or more and then shipped on the Barcelona packet, an inter-insular trading ship. He worked four or five days, after which he fell sick with a fever which shortly proved fatal.

Upon arrival at his home port several months later Captain Paul was met with a warrant filed by Maxwell's father charging murder of the son. After a long wait necessary for the assembling of evidence the accusation was rejected by the court as groundless, but the animosity of the home folks toward the upstart Captain could not be rescinded by law. Among the sailors, dock-wallopers, and water-front riff-raff at Tobago the incident was likewise well remembered. So, when in 1773 John Paul returned to Tobago port in charge of another trader and there ran his sword through a sailor who, it is said, was pursuing and menacing him with an axe, there was no safety thereabouts for Captain Paul. He surrendered promptly to a local magistrate. Though himself convinced that it was a clear case of self-defense, the magistrate was obliged to refer the case to the Admiralty Court, which would not sit at Tobago for some months. Accordingly Paul was released on his promise to present himself before the high court in due season. The delicate question confronting the defendant was, what to do meantime? The island of Tobago was seething with men who would enjoy nothing more than slitting the throat of an arrogant sea captain. Paul's friends, among whom was Mr. William Young, lieutenant governor of the island of Tobago, advised him to leave the vicinity at once. In token of their sincerity his advisers presented him with a horse and a purse of fifty pounds, whereupon the Captain headed his steed toward a far side of the little island that very night and disappeared in the darkness.

As a boy apprentice on the brig *Friendship*, John Paul had visited the shores of Virginia and is known to have had an older brother, William Paul, at Fredericksburg. It was therefore no mere coincidence that two years after the Tobago homicide a man bearing all the physical attributes of Captain John Paul turned up at, or in the vicinity of, Fredericksburg. At first he called himself John P. Jones, but shortly he was known as John Paul Jones.

Through his friendship with Dr. John Read, a well-known Virginia physician whom he seems to have met casually, Jones became acquainted with Washington, Jefferson, the Lees, and other influential persons in Virginia Colony who supported his ambitions for an active role when the storms of war struck. In 1779, Jones seems to have cleared up the mystery of his name pretty well when he wrote his good friend, Benjamin Franklin, that it had been his honest intention to return to Tobago for trial, but the onset of the Colonial Revolution rendered the plan unfeasible, adding that it was the advice of the acting governor of the island and other friends that he should "return incog. to the continent of America."

There has been much speculation as to how and where Jones spent the twenty-odd months between the Tobago episode and his appearance in Virginia. Since he seemed disinclined to talk about it, many persons have construed his reticence to mean that he was engaged in some sort of dark business. It is known that the Tobago homicide weighed heavily on his conscience for many years and that he was not the kind to engage in murder or other gross violation of the fundamental laws of civilized men. His best defense, however, is his subsequent record of loyal, humane, and distinguished service to the country to which he had pledged his allegiance.

It is known that in his youth he worked for a time on a slave trader plying the seas between Africa and Jamaica and that he quit his job in disgust. It must be admitted, however, that the "severe fevers," probably malarial, which plagued him at the time, may have heightened his repugnance for that sort of traffic. A few years later while engaged in the West India trade he had chronic malaria as, indeed, did all others similarly employed. On the whole, however, his health up to his middle thirties seems to have been about as good as the average of those in his environment. Physically he was not large, but he was compactly built and he had the smooth-working, resilient muscles of a feline. Russell gives this description of Jones as he appeared when about the age of thirty:

"From his slender legs his body stems gracefully outward to a pair of powerful shoulders, roomy chest, and a swart, thickish neck. Moving with a pronounced dignity, he appears to be a formidable figure; and yet there is only five feet seven inches of him. His mouth is soft though a little hard at the ends. His hands and feet are small like a girl's. As he approaches the ship it is seen that his powdered hair, tied with a queue at the back, is really a dark brown and that his straight gazing, restless black eyes are really a dark grey formed between jutting cheek bones."

While he was engaged in outfitting the *Bonhomme Richard*, Jones was stricken with a severe illness, the nature of which is not known but is ascribed by his biographers to "disappointment, lack of sleep, and worry." As the attack came suddenly in the spring of the year and seems to have been febrile in character, we may conjecture that he suffered a recurrence of the malaria which infested his system while he was in the West Indies. He was not the type of young man to let disappointment get him down. In his middle thirties, however, he began to complain openly of ill health; he coughed a great deal and he had frequent attacks of bronchitis. Evidently he had at this time a chronic asthma of the subclinical type, a continuing engorgement of the finer bronchial ramifications (bronchioles), usually called bronchiolitis and readily diagnosable by auscultation and forced expiration. Bronchiolitis conduces to frequent coughs and colds such as troubled Jones the remainder of his life. It may be due to extrinsic causes (allergy) or it may be due to some unknown intrinsic factor. The first type is usually curable, the second type is often incurable. Both types, if permitted to run on, tend to become frank, clinical asthma.

In 1783 Jones lived in London for a time where he was engaged in the highly profitable business of buying cargoes of whale oil and selling them in France and Holland. He is reported to have recouped a substantial percentage of the personal losses he had sustained during the war. A lengthy sojourn in a rest home improved his health considerably and, for a fleeting moment, fortune seems to have smiled upon the long-suffering commander. He left England for Paris, where he succeeded in obtaining a small partial payment from the French government for prizes taken during the war. It should be borne in mind that Jones' claims were not made primarily on his own account; mostly they were made in behalf of the men who served under him and who, like their commander, had not been paid the wages so perilously earned.

From France, Jones again returned to the United States and

presented his claims against the United States Treasury. The Board of Treasury admitted the validity of his claims but pleaded inability to pay the whole amount. The claimant scorned anything less than full payment, and on November 11, 1787, departed for France, never again to set foot upon the land for which he had offered his life and sacrificed most of his worldly possessions. But he did not leave our shores empty handed; the Congress awarded him a gold medal before he got away, commemorating his services to the nation when it was a-borning. Fifty-six years after his death the claim was paid to two female relatives who, so the court held, were the legal heirs to the Jones estate.

Upon his arrival in France he proceeded at once to his old haunts in Paris. There he received the astonishing news that Catherine II wished him to come to Russia to enter her service against the Turks. But Jones desired first of all to make a settlement with the Danes for three war prizes which the Danish government had illegally restored to England. He arrived at Copenhagen ill and exhausted. He was having another of his frequent "bad colds." His mission to Denmark having failed of its purpose, he reluctantly accepted Catherine's invitation and set out for St. Petersburg. The treatment he experienced at the Russian capital indicates that Russian character has changed very little since the eighteenth century. It seems likely that he never would have escaped from the country alive but for the vigorous intervention of the French ambassador in his behalf. So, instead of having him assassinated as she probably was planning to do, Catherine made him a rear admiral and gave him a two-years' leave of absence with pay. Her strategy, it is supposed, was to play upon his sense of loyalty to her Majesty and thereby restrain him from going over to the side of the Swedes or some other enemy of her empire. Secretly she denounced him as "a thoroughly bad person," but *she did pay him his salary*.

"Admiral" Jones returned to Paris in May, 1790, weary, sick, and dejected, but not disillusioned. He still entertained the preposterous notion that he was fit for sea duty and he continued to dream of himself in command of a powerful fleet fighting victoriously in the cause of righteousness. Although he was only forty-three, his hair was graying, he looked old and shrunken, and he coughed and wheezed incessantly. It was commonly believed that he had pulmonary tuberculosis.

Early in July, 1792, Gouverneur Morris, United States ambassador to France, visited Jones in his apartment and reported him "extremely cheerful and seemed better than for a long time previously. He did not cough much and talked a good deal." Despite the Minister's optimism, the Commander's condition worsened daily. On July 11 his legs were noticeably swollen; by the morning of the eighteenth the swelling was much more intense and had extended to the lower abdomen. On the evening of the same day he was last seen alive, sitting in an armchair in his quarters. Some time during the night of July 18–19, with the French Revolution breaking around him, John Paul Jones toddled to his bed, fell face down upon it, and, with his toes touching the floor, expired.

Ambassador Morris was too busy with social affairs to be bothered with funeral arrangements for one who had been so unimportant socially as the dead commander, but the King's commisary and the National Assembly of France united to give the remains a proper ceremonial interment. The body was placed in a lead coffin and buried in the St. Louis Protestant Cemetery. Then the event was forgotten and the cemetery likewise when it became overspread by the creeping squalor of Paris' *bas quartiers*. In 1899, however, General Horace Porter, United States ambassador to France, learned that a slum-clearance project was about to uncover the little Protestant cemetery and, at his own expense, undertook to locate the body of Jones. Three weeks of exploration disclosed five lead coffins, one of which certainly contained the remains of the Commander. By a meticulous process of elimination a body conforming in all preservable detail to that of Jones was found. It was in remarkably good condition. There was no evidenced that it had been embalmed, but a strong odor of alcohol indicated that the corpse had been saturated with some sort of spiritous solution. Certificates were signed by French and American officials alike, affirming their faith in the correctness of the identification.[1]

[1] As might be expected, the verdict of the officials has not met with universal acceptance.

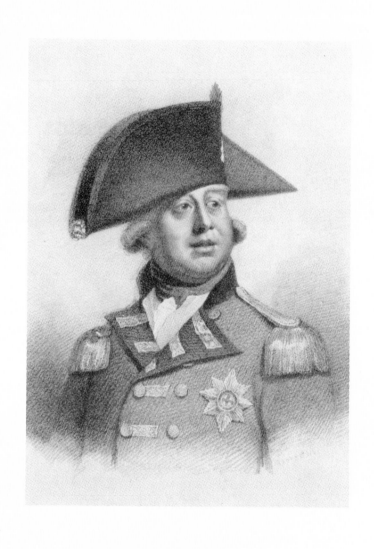

GEORGE III

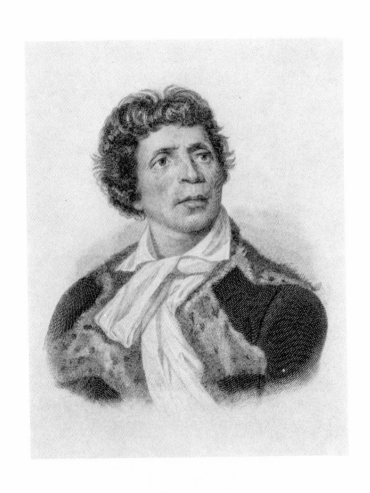

JEAN PAUL MARAT

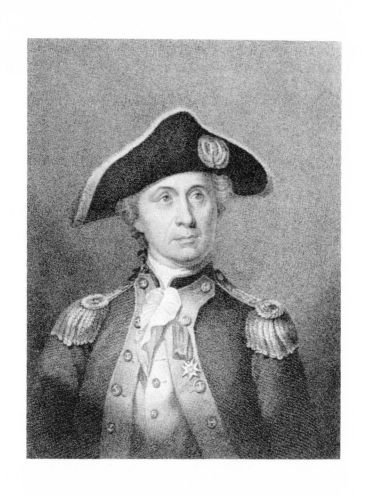

JOHN PAUL JONES

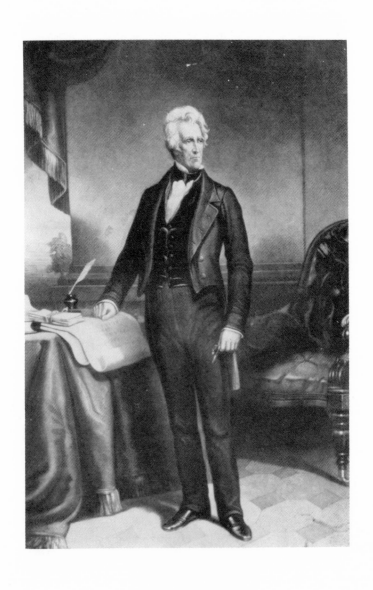

ANDREW JACKSON

Of particular importance in establishing the identity of the body was the aid rendered by two distinguished French scientists from the Paris School of Anthropology. They were Dr. G. Papillant, who confirmed the identification on the basis of known physical characteristics of the Commander, and Dr. J. Capitan, who dissected the body. The autopsy, which was performed on April 13, 1905, has been somewhat ambiguously described as "the oldest autopsy in history." It is of great interest because of the light it throws upon the cause of Jones' ill health and death, and because it was made 113 years after decease. Dr. Capitan's report is quoted:

"In order not to alter in any way the appearance of the corpse, I made the autopsy by opening the back. Upon opening the thorax I was greatly astonished to find the viscera much contracted but very well preserved. The lungs presented some adhesions to the pleural walls, especially in the upper lobes. When cut open they show a brownish parenchyma. Upon the surface and in the interior of the pulmonary tissue there exists, especially at the level of the diaphragmatic edge of the lower lobe, small white hard masses 3 to 4 millimeters in diameter, and having the appearance of calcified tubercles. But in view of the existence of concretions of an analagous appearance at the surface of the teguments of the lower limbs, this diagnosis cannot be sustained. Besides, as will be seen, it is a question of a mass of tyrosin. . . .

"The liver was yellowish brown. The gallbladder was healthy and contained a pale yellowish bile of a pasty consistency. The stomach was very small and contracted. The spleen appeared comparatively more voluminous than it ought to have been, considering the marked contraction of all the viscera. The two kidneys were small, hard, and contracted. The intestines were completely contracted and empty. The head was not opened."

Miscroscopic examination revealed that ". . . the heart is normal with streaks of some muscular fibers still very clearly visible. The liver seems likewise normal. It was not possible to see whether there had been such cellular lesions as accompany the acute liver troubles analogous to symptoms of jaundice which Paul Jones presented at the end of his life. The lungs contain in sufficiently large numbers these white granulations which seem to have, under the microscope, the appearance of fine needles of tyrosin [product of the decomposition of azotized substances]. The presence of these crystals can be explained, as before the alcohol could have penetrated all the viscera there took place a beginning of decomposition which brought on the production of the crystals."

With respect to the lungs, "The only lesions that one could locate were small rounded masses, hard and at times calcified in the lungs, which correspond to small patches of broncho-pneumonia partially cicatrized. . . .

"As to the kidneys, the sections presented the appearance of chronic interstitial nephritis. The vessels at several points had their walls thickened and invaded by sclerosis. A number of glomeruli were completely transformed into fibrous tissue and appeared in the form of small spheres."

Dr. Capitan concluded that the body was that of John Paul Jones and that death was due to broncho-pneumonia and "chronic pyelonephritis." Certain comments seem proper: First of all, the autopsy findings may be said to have contributed to the identification of the body to the extent that the broncho-pneumonia was perfectly consistent with the symptoms which for several weeks had preceded death, and the enlarged spleen (ague cake) was an inevitable sequence of the severe and prolonged malarial infection he had suffered on the African coast and later in the West Indies. But the kidney pathology was quite unexpected and is not easily explained. The description given by Dr. Capitan indicates that Jones suffered from what is now called "glomerular nephritis," the cause of which, in general, is not yet well understood. The best guess in the Jones case, however, is that it came from the intense respiratory tract infection and had its beginning in the hardships he endured on his way to Russia in 1788.

Dr. Capitan's statement that on microscopic examination "the heart is *normal* with *some* muscular fibers still clearly visible" is very confusing. Certainly a heart so far gone with post-mortem changes that merely *some* of the fibers are visible cannot be said to be "normal" in the sense that pre-mortem disease processes have been excluded. As the dropsical condition from which the Commander suffered in the last few weeks of his life involved only the dependent parts of the body, it was not the edema of acute nephritis. Rather, it was due to a decompensated heart which had resulted from the high blood pressure incidental to chronic glomer-ular nephritis. Clinically, he died a cardiac death.

By way of postscript, it may be recounted that in 1905, in the course of some vigorous drum-beating for a larger navy, President Theodore Roosevelt directed Admiral Charles D. Sigsbee to proceed to France with a naval squadron for the purpose of bringing Jones' remains to the United States. Accompanied by an honorary escort of French war vessels, the United States cruisers brought the casketed body of the Commander to Annapolis where it was placed in a brick vault on the Naval Academy grounds. On April 24, 1906, impressive memorial exercises were held at the Academy, in the course of which stirring addresses were made by President Roosevelt, French Ambassador Jusserand, and other notables. After "the tumult and the fury" died and the speakers and the listeners had departed, the body of the much-lauded hero was carried to Bancroft Hall and placed on two wooden saw-horses. There it rested for seven years before, in response to public agitation, it was placed in the handsome tomb beneath the naval chapel where it now lies.

Perhaps after all, republics are *not* ungrateful; *not* in the long, long run.

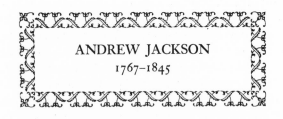

HE MEDICAL LIFE of the seventh president of the United States is a song of valor and an epic of fortitude. Certainly no other of our national heroes has had to contend against the mass and variety of enemies that tortured the body but could not conquer the spirit of the dauntless General Jackson of Tennessee.

Andrew, the third son of Andrew Jackson and Elizabeth Hutchinson Jackson, was born in the Waxhaw Settlement of South Carolina a few days after his father died, allegedly from the exertions of attempting to lift a fallen tree. Most accounts agree that the place of birth was the James Crawford plantation, but others argue that the momentous event occurred at the home of George McKemey. The discrepancy is important principally because the present state line, which has separated the Carolinas since 1813, passes between the sites of the two habitations. Wherefore, with each state insistently claiming the General for its own, no man can safely say he has seen the birthplace of Andrew Jackson unless he has visited both spots and honored both claimants.

As a young lad, Andy was not of prepossessing appearance. At the age of fourteen he was a tall, skinny, sandy-haired, freckled-faced fledgling whose general homeliness was alleviated only by a pair of intensely blue eyes. From childhood through adolescence he had a pronounced tendency to drool when he talked, especially if excited, a peculiarity which brought many taunts and approximately the same number of fights. No matter what the odds against him, Andrew could be depended upon to give battle instantly if he was slighted, defied, or insulted.

Before he was fourteen years of age, Andy had smelled the smoke of battle in a skirmish or two with the British and the Tories. And on April 9, 1781, when he had turned fourteen by less than a month, he was captured by a body of dragoons who descended upon the home of his cousin, Lieutenant Crawford, where Andrew and several other rebels were having breakfast. His brother, Robert Jackson, aged sixteen, was taken with him. Immediately following the capture a British subaltern who was in command of the raiders ordered Andrew, "in a very imperious tone," to clean his boots. This task the impertinent lad refused to perform. The officer swung his sword. Andy threw up his left hand to ward off the blow and received a deep wound on the wrist and a gash in the side of the head. Robert, equally defiant, received wounds of a more serious nature.

Following their capture the two brothers were imprisoned at Camden, where shortly both came down with smallpox. Spirited Elizabeth Jackson, learning of the plight of her two sons, rode a horse forty miles to Camden, where she went before the commanding officer and negotiated the release of the two sick lads. A horse was procured for the desperately sick Robert, but Andrew walked, alternately clinging to a stirrup and to the tail of one of the animals for support and traction. The effort of the journey combined with exposure to chilling rain was too much for Robert, who died two days after reaching home. Andrew barely survived the trip and his smallpox to lie helpless for weeks with chills and fever. In a country where almost everyone carried the Plasmodium in his system, any sort of intercurrent fever was likely to activate a dormant malaria. Andrew's malaria was the aftermath of his smallpox.

As soon as Andrew appeared to be out of danger, his mother with a number of other women of the neighborhood set out to nurse certain local boys who were sick with "ship fever" in a floating prison which Cornwallis had established off Charles Town. The term "ship fever" is one of several outmoded names for deadly typhus fever. A few weeks before Christmas Andrew received a bundle of clothes and belongings which he recognized only too

137

well. Elizabeth Jackson had been buried along with other victims of the plague on the dismal flat of Charles Town Neck.

When he was about sixteen, Andrew received a legacy of three or four hundred pounds sterling from the estate of his grandfather, Hugh Jackson, of Carrickfergus which is an old town on the northern coast of Ireland near Belfast. For many generations it was the home of Andrew Jackson's forefathers. It was on a March day in 1783 that the young legatee stepped out of the Quarter House Tavern in Charles Town with enough money in his pocket to make a neat estate out of the old family homestead or to pay for two or three years' schooling. But he got home with neither part nor parcel of his easy-come fortune. As the principal business of that section of the country at the time appears to have been horse racing, Andrew's reversion to impecuniousness may, perhaps, be called a case of "business failure." At any rate his brief role of young gentleman is said to have stimulated him to seek an education, wherefore it may be considered a moral gain. After a short term in school he felt he should turn his newly acquired knowledge to some account, and the pupil became teacher. But the atmosphere of pedagogy was too stuffy for one of his restive and competitive temperament. The profession of law seemed more to his liking, and he therefore attached himself to Attorney Spruce Macay, who let him read law in the Macay office. Gossip has it that after a year Macay was displeased with Andrew's general behavior and refused to sponsor the entrance of so wild a character into the honorable calling which he himself so nobly represented. But with the aid of another attorney who possessed a good law library and an indulgent attitude of mind, Andrew was able to scale the ramparts of respectability and enter the circle of the elect. On September 27, 1728, at the age of twenty-one and one-half years, Andrew Jackson, "a person of unblemished moral character," was admitted to the practice of law "with all and singular the privileges and emoluments which pertain to attorneys."

In October he moved to Nashville, where he was installed as prosecutor in the court of Judge John McNairy. Unable to find suitable lodgings in the city, Lawyer Jackson took up his abode at Widow Donelson's blockhouse, a full ten miles in the country. The place was not easy of access, but if at first Jackson had any idea of seeking more conveniently located quarters later, the plan fell apart after he had his first good look at his landlady's attractive daughter.

Rachel Donelson Robards, having married into a well-to-do family and made a pious but futile effort to get along with a completely unreasonable husband, took the first recourse of a harassed daughter; she came home to mother. Return to the maternal fireside had preceded the arrival of the young attorney by only a few weeks. It seems likely that as the days passed, Jackson, in the courtly manner which he reserved exclusively for the benefit of ladies, had made Rachel aware of his interest in her. But she had not taken her marriage vows lightly and when a penitent husband sought reconciliation, it was granted. It endured only a few months. This time Robards took the initiative and left Rachel. On December 20, 1790, the Virginia Assembly passed a bill granting Robards the right to sue for divorce in the state of Kentucky, which was then in the process of cleavage from the mother state. He did not follow through, so that when Andrew and Rachel were married in August, 1791, in the comfortable belief that no legal impediment existed, they were grievously mistaken. Robards waited until September 27, 1793, to get his divorce. It was granted on evidence that Rachel had deserted her lawful husband and "hath and doth still, live in adultery with another man." Jackson has been criticized with some justice for his failure to ascertain Rachel's status under the law before leading her into another marriage. There was a second marriage ceremony after the illegality of the first had been disclosed. But the tongues of scandal continued to wag.

Andrew was a fiercely devoted husband ever ready with cane, horsewhip, or pistol to defend the character of his wife against any and all calumniators. One of his battles in defense of Rachel's chastity nearly cost him his life. When he heard that his racing rival, aristocratic young Charles Dickinson, had made disrespectful allusion to Rachel's matrimonial record, Jackson promptly confronted him and demanded an apology. Dickinson asked pardon, explaining that he was drunk at the time he spoke the hateful words. Soon, however, Jackson learned that the offense had been repeated. As always happens when a good fight foreshadows, there was no lack of partisans to egg on the disputants. Dickinson dared Jackson to challenge and received a prompt acceptance. Seconds were chosen, details agreed upon, and arrangements made.

Dickinson was an expert pistol shot, which is to say, in the language of the idiom, he could shoot both fast and straight. Jackson, aware of Dickinson's vastly superior marksmanship, decided that it was useless to try to beat him to the first fire. Instead he resolved grimly to survive the expected hit long enough to kill his adversary. It was agreed that the duel should be fought a few miles above the border in Kentucky on May 30, 1806. Jackson chafed at the long wait of one week and protested the forty-mile ride made as a gesture of respect for Tennessee's defunct anti-dueling law.

On the evening of May 29, Jackson with his second, General Thomas Overton, arrived at Miller's Tavern, Kentucky, about eight o'clock. Nothing could better illustrate the iron nerve of the man than Jackson's behavior the night before the fateful contest. After supper he sat chatting with other guests on the porch of the inn. No one suspected the purpose of the journey. At ten o'clock he knocked the dottle from his pipe and went to bed. In ten minutes he was asleep, and at five the next morning it was necessary to rouse him.

At sunrise the parties met in a clearing in a poplar woods on the bank of Red River. Dickinson's second was a Dr. Catlett. The weapons belonged to Jackson, but Dickinson was permitted to take his choice of the two identical pistols. Each was of seventy caliber with a nine-inch barrel loaded with a one-ounce lead ball. The distance was twenty-four feet and, as stipulated in the written agreement, "the parties to stand facing each other with their pistols down perpendicularly. When they are Ready, the single word, Fire! to be given at which they are to fire as soon as they please."

The distance was paced off and the principals took their stance. Jackson wore a loose-fitting frock coat with trousers to match; Dickinson a short coat of blue with gray trousers. General Overton called, "Gentlemen, you are ready?" "Ready," said Dickinson. "Yes, sir," said Jackson. " 'Fere!' shouted Overton in the old-country accent."[1]

Dickinson fired instantly, without seeming to aim. He had promised to shoot Jackson through the heart. Jackson's left hand clutched his chest. He did not stagger, but seemed momentarily stunned. Regaining control of himself he slowly raised his pistol. Dickinson retreated a step, his face pale as he exclaimed, "Great God! Have I missed him?" Overton pointed his pistol and ordered, "Back to the mark, sir!" Dickinson stepped to the line and stood with folded arms, his eyes averted. Jackson took aim and pulled the trigger of his weapon. The hammer stopped at half-cock. He drew it to full cock and aimed again. This time it fired. Dickinson swayed and fell to the ground.

As Jackson and Overton strode to their horses, the second noticed blood on Jackson's left boot, but the victim made light of his injury. Subsequently it was revealed that Dickinson's bullet had shattered a couple of ribs and entered Jackson's chest to the left of the heart. At the crucial instant the loser had forgotten to make allowance for the narrowness of his adversary's chest. Dickinson, his entrails torn by the heavy slug, died after sixteen hours of unmitigated agony.

Jackson was confined to his bed for a month. The doctors said the bullet lay dangerously near the heart and the wounded man should lie quietly for many more weeks. But no sooner had Nature restored the lost blood sufficiently than the patient rose from his bed to launch an inquiry into the allegedly treasonable designs of his friend, Aaron Burr.

It seems very probable that the bullet which Jackson carried in his chest the rest of his life did not lie as close to the heart as the doctors believed. Persons of Jackson's build have "drop heart," which is to say, the chest being extremely long and narrow, the organ of circulation lies lower than in persons of heavy or medium physique and the long axis assumes an approximately vertical direction. In stocky individuals the direction of the long axis approximates the horizontal and in persons of ordinary build it usually lies

[1] Somewhat conflicting accounts are given with respect to the stipulations and particulars of the duel. The version given here is essentially that of Marquis James.

about midway between these two extremes. Almost surely the ball lay not only to the left of the heart but above it as well. Mr. Dickinson might have profited from a knowledge of anatomy.

The duel with Dickinson marked a turning point in the health of Andrew Jackson. Up to his fortieth year his portion of illness probably had not been much greater than that of the average person of that age in a community where all the commoner contagious diseases raged unchecked and malarial infection was universal. But from the year of the fateful affair of honor with Charles Dickinson, his biography is dotted with references to cough, hemorrhages from the lungs, intermittent fever, chills and fever, and attacks of dysentery. Undoubtedly some of these bouts of fever were due to malaria, but most of them were occasioned by an abscess within his chest centering about the bullet so ceremoniously introduced by Mr. Dickinson. Sometimes the abscess cavity was sealed off, giving rise to "low fever" merging into chills with sharp rises of temperature. Eventually the accumulated pus, following a fistulous track, which closed off between times, would break through into a bronchial tube. Severe cough with expectoration of blood and pus ensued. His condition seemed acutely critical at the time, but actually it was like the negative phase following a surgical operation. Relieved of his sepsis, the sick man convalesced with astounding rapidity. So went the cycle year after year. The pulmonary bleeding gave rise to the belief that Jackson had pulmonary tuberculosis, the contagion which had decimated his wife's family. It can be stated with considerable confidence that Jackson did not have tuberculosis.

As for the dysentery, it undoubtedly was that and not simple diarrhoea. Whether it was of the amoebic or the bacillary type is impossible to say, though the factor of relative frequency would favor the latter. As everyone knows, few ailments are better designed to rob life of its purpose and impress the mind with a sense of complete futility than the double-barreled affliction of cramps and diarrhoea. But it couldn't stop General Jackson or deflect him in the slightest from the pursuit of his historic objectives. Apparently he contracted his dysentery shortly after he took the field in the war against the Creek Indians. For the next decade his biography records many and severe visitations of diarrhoea in all sorts of places and circumstances. But in no instance is it recorded that he surrendered to the disease and "laid up" when there was work to be done.

On September 4, 1813, at the City Hotel in Nashville, Jackson pulled a pistol on Tom Benton for what would seem to be trivial reasons and was fired upon from behind by Benton's brother, Jesse. One of the two bullets with which Jesse's pistol was loaded struck Jackson's left upper arm near the shoulder joint, smashed the bone (humerus), and lodged at the site of wreckage. The other is commonly said to have shattered the shoulder, but study of the medical evidence warrants the conclusion that Jackson was hit by only one of the two missiles. Perhaps confusion has arisen from failure to appreciate the anatomical fact that the upper extremity of the humerus is an integral part of the shoulder.

At the Nashville Inn where Jackson was taken immediately after the shooting, he bled so profusely that two mattresses are said to have been ruined by the outpour. Every doctor in Nashville came to his aid, and all but one advised amputation without delay, but the exsanguinated General whispered, "I'll keep my arm." Before partisans of the two principals could take up the quarrel, news came of the massacre at Fort Mims by Creek Indians and the winds of belligerence changed their direction. The governor of Mississippi Territory authorized an expedition of twenty-five hundred men. As James remarks, "Jackson was too weak to leave his bed but he was strong enough to make war." He promised the governor that he would be ready to take command in nine days. Knowing well the weaknesses of the civilian contract-supply system then in vogue, the General appealed to the people of Mississippi, saying, "There is an enemy I dread much more than I do the hostile Creek . . . that meager monster, famine." The Indians were badly beaten in two battles by the General with the mangled arm, to whose discomfort had been added an attack of dysentery. During paroxysms of rapidly recurring cramps, he sometimes draped his body over a "sapling half severed and bent over," remaining in this least-uncomfortable position for hours at a time. The pressure exerted against the abdomen had a splint-like effect on the writhing intestines and thus gave a modicum of relief from the pain. "That meager monster" did appear and threatened to rob the General of the fruits of his two victories over the savage enemy. With the campaign stalled for lack of food, the few remaining beeves were given to the men while the commander and his staff ate the viscera without bread or salt. However, despite famine, governmental cowardice, rebellious troops, and constant physical distress, the iron-willed General brought the campaign to a victorious conclusion.

In 1814, while waiting at Mobile en route to New Orleans, Jackson's unhealed left arm sloughed a fragment of bone. He sent the grim token of mortality to Rachel with romantic sentiments of love. In December, 1815, he arrived, wracked by dysentery, at the outskirts of New Orleans, looking as if he were freshly disinterred. At an elaborate breakfast prepared in his honor by a prominent citizen, the General passed up a gourmet's phantasy for a few spoonfuls of hominy and a glass of milk. Some evenings later at a reception given in his honor by the city officials, he was so spick, span, and resplendent in his attire and so suave, gallant, and proper in his manners that all those present gasped in astonished admiration. General Jackson was like that.

After New Orleans and the end of hostilities came return to the Hermitage and horses. His health was good in a relative sense only. Chills, diarrhoea, and cough with expectoration of blood were noted in the records from time to time. During his few months' tenure of the governorship of Florida his health declined, and after he returned home in the autumn of 1821, he suffered from a "distressing cough and inflammation of the lungs." He decided that he was getting old and should "be done with public life." In 1822 he caught a severe cold to which was added the old "bowell complaint which has weakened me much . . . having in the last twelve hours upward of twenty passages. . . . In short, Sir, I must take a rest or my stay on Erth cannot be long." Just preceding the severe cold and the recurrence of the "bowell" complaint, there was a protracted spell of costiveness associated with severe cramps. It is more than possible that his costiveness and cramps were due to lead poisoning. When we reflect that an ordinary twenty-two caliber bullet weighing not more than forty grains may, if lying beneath the skin, cause a fatal lead poisoning, it seems incredible that Jackson who harbored a 480-grain leaden slug in his chest and another in his left arm could have escaped some degree of plumbism. If more than two ounces of lead was necessary, it may have been supplied by his habitual use of sugar of lead (lead acetate) for practically all his ailments, whether internal or external. He bathed his eyes with a solution of sugar of lead, he poured it into his wounds to insure prompt healing, and he even drank it for his intestinal cramps.

On December 17, 1828, Rachel Jackson suffered a heart attack, the symptoms and termination of which were typical for coronary thrombosis. For three days she lay in unspeakable agony; then the pain began to abate and by dawn of the sixth day she was fairly comfortable. On the evening of that day she was assisted to a chair, where she sat while the bed was being made. Suddenly, as she sat, she uttered an inarticulate cry, her head fell forward on her chest and she was gone. The desolate husband, unable to comprehend the fact of her death, had her body placed on four blankets spread on a table and sat beside it throughout the night watching for respiratory movements that did not appear and feeling for a pulse that would not return. Only six weeks previously Andrew had been made President-elect of the United States. Poor Rachel, who neither knew nor aspired to know anything of elegant society, was appalled by contemplation of her prospective social responsibilities. Perhaps her death at this time was, after all, a kindly intervention of Providence, for it saved her from the certain sneers and slanders which would have lacerated her sensitive soul had she lived to be mistress of the White House.

During his first year as chief executive, Jackson's legs were swollen much of the time and a fatal attack of dropsy was feared. It did not seem possible that anyone in his condition could live through a four-year term in the Presidency. Remarkably, he not only survived but even regained some of his old fighting form after a visiting surgeon from Philadelphia removed Jesse Benton's bullet from the crippled arm. Had the operation been of the emergency type, it could scarcely have been done with greater dispatch. The patient bared the arm and took a firm grip on his walking stick. The surgeon gashed the skin and popped the bullet out. It is claimed that there was a prompt improvement in the President's health. If so, it was due, in all probability, to amelioration of the bone infection (osteomyelitis) which must have been aggravated by the presence of the foreign body during its nineteen years' residence in the damaged arm.

In 1833 while visiting in Philadelphia, the President was examined by Dr. Philip Syng Physick, whose glory rested not in his name but in his skill as a surgeon. Dr. Physick was so captivated by the keen intelligence and the friendly and forthright manner of his distinguished patient that he was loath to talk of anything else for several days afterward. For the chronic pain in the side, due to a pleuritis caused by extension of inflammation from the abscessed area surrounding Charles Dickinson's bullet, the doctor advised cupping. It was as good a remedy as the medical knowledge of the times afforded, but it gave little relief. When, continuing his junket, the President entered Boston, the town was prepared to be coolly receptive. Rarely indeed has that staid city been so happily shaken from its resolute complacency. On the second day Josiah Quincy, president of Harvard College, called his overseers together and obtained permission to confer the degree of Doctor of Laws upon the backwoodsman from Tennessee. Only John Quincy Adams, jealous of his Alma Mater's record of scholastic purity, raised his voice in vigorous but futile protest against the award.

During the week in Boston, Jackson was bedfast for two days with an acute cold and the night before his departure for Salem he suffered a severe pulmonary hemorrhage. At Salem he was put to bed under a doctor's care. But despite stresses, strains, and breakdowns, when he returned to the White House after twenty-seven days of political adventuring, he seemed definitely better than when he set out.

During his second term his health was, if possible, worse than during the first term. At any rate, he found it necessary to curb his physical activities more than ever before. About four months before he was due to take his final leave of Washington, he suffered another severe attack of cough and hemorrhage. His doctors demonstrated the indestructibility of their patient by promptly letting nearly two quarts of his blood. Forty-eight hours later he was sitting up. When Jackson's tenure of office expired in March, 1837, his successor, Martin Van Buren, tried to dissuade him from leaving until he had taken a few days' rest. But his impatience to be back at the Hermitage was so acute that he could not have rested if he had consented to stay. President Van Buren directed Dr. John Laws, surgeon general of the army, to accompany the Jackson party as far as Wheeling. There other army doctors took over and remained with the former President until he was safely home. The following October a visitor to the Hermitage found the old General in his shirt sleeves waiting by the roadside for the mail coach while a chill wind swept about his meager frame. He would not take care of himself. At this time it was noted that his right eye was almost blind, probably from the encroachment of a pterygium upon the pupil, and his mind seemed to lack its former alertness.

Precisely what caused the swelling of the legs, first noted in 1829, can never be surely known. Apparently the condition subsided and recurred a number of times until the last two or three years of his life, when it became chronic and grew slowly worse with the passing months. In the beginning it may have been caused by severe anemia resulting from chronic infection, pulmonary hemorrhages, and the senseless letting of blood. Swelling of the legs is often observed in ambulant cases of high-grade anemia whether of the primary or secondary type. One thing seems clear: the dropsical condition of the legs in 1829 was not a result of heart disease. A heart once broken down does not, in the absence of enlightened medical care, carry on for the next seventeen years as Jackson's heart did.

Gardner ascribes "the grisly last years of the patient and miserable sufferer" to amyloidosis, a term applied to depositions of a peculiar protein substance, with a starchlike reaction to iodine stain, in various organs of the body, especially the kidneys, liver, and spleen. Apart from the rare primary type, amyloidosis is found almost exclusively in persons suffering from chronic suppurative disease or advanced tuberculosis, usually of the pulmonary type, with cavitation. It is true that Jackson had a chronic pulmonary abscess of the left lung, probably with associated bronchiectasis (dilated bronchial tubes) of both lungs[2] and also an osteomyelitis, a proper set-up for the production of amyloidosis. But amyloido-

[2] If one of the lungs is involved in a chronic purulent process, the

sis is generally regarded as only as important as its underlying cause. When amyloid kidney disease is associated with dropsy, the latter is due partly to the anemia caused by the basic chronic infection and partly to loss by way of the amyloid kidney of great quantities of proteins essential for the maintenance of normal blood viscosity. The watery blood plasma seeps through the vessel walls and accumulates in the adjacent tissues to produce the boggy swelling of dependent portions of the body characteristic of the dropsical state. Amyloidosis is unrelated to true nephritis. Typically the blood pressure is below normal levels and the pulse has a double-beat or dicrotic quality. The patient presents a picture of extreme malnutrition and debility. In these days of surgical competency and antibiotic drugs the condition is extremely rare. It probably was not very common even in the days when chronic suppurative disease and instances of far-advanced pulmonary tuberculosis were to be found in almost every village in the land.

Contrary to Gardner's assertion, medical authorities do not consider amyloidosis "implacable." Removal of the causal factor usually results in improvement and sometimes in clinical cure of well-established cases of amyloidosis. In the case of Jackson, amyloidosis may have been present to some extent during the last few years of his life. But when a septuagenarian who has endured lung abscess, cough, fever, pulmonary hemorrhages, osteomyelitis, and periodic diarrhoea for thirty-odd years finally begins to falter, it would seem unnecessary to search the fringes of morbidity in order to find a reasonable explanation for his decrepitude.

A sore trial for Jackson was his foster-son, Andrew Jackson, Jr. The boy was a nephew of Rachel, who had carried him home with her when a frail sister-in-law found herself unequipped by nature to suckle her twin boys born in December, 1810. Junior grew up, it seems, his soul completely uncontaminated by the vulgar profit motive. Trusted with care of the Hermitage and management of the plantation during his father's absence in Washington, he made foolish commitments and signed as surety on so many bad debts that poor old Andrew, who disdained the refuge

bronchial tubes of the opposite lung become inflamed as a result of inhalation of infected material.

of bankruptcy for the boy, was actually impoverished in the last years of his life. Altogether he spent an estimated forty thousand dollars settling his son's bad accounts. How much more was lost through unproductive crop management cannot be estimated.

Early in 1838 the ailing General had planned to visit one of Tennessee's several "healing springs," but was forced to cancel the project because of a lack of necessary cash. He found solace, however, in a nostrum called "Matchless Sanative" which, he declared, was "making a new man" out of him. For some years he kept a bottle of the matchless elixir always at hand and publicly extolled its virtues as a remedy for pulmonary complaints. It appears that the formula is lost to posterity.

In January, 1840, he accepted an invitation to visit New Orleans in commemoration of his great victory over the British twenty-five years before. His health was so poor that he preferred staying at home, but it was necessary to secure modification of the terms under which Andrew, Jr., had purchased Halcyon Plantation in Mississippi some years before. In the course of the journey the old General could conveniently stop off and plead his case before young Andrew's creditors. Despite severe hemorrhages, extreme weakness, and shortness of breath, he managed to survive the ten days and nights of receptions, banquets, and speeches; and, importantly, he obtained the sought-for concessions from the Halcyon mortgagees. It was his last long trip.

The resilient thread of life may be stretched to amazing lengths before it breaks. When Jackson left the White House in 1837, no one could have believed he would live for eight years thereafter. Yet live he did, despite the aggravated state of his old ailments and the acquisition of a few new ones. Early in 1845 when each breath he drew seemed likely to be his last, one of his ailments turned against another; he suddenly developed a severe watery diarrhoea which drained away his dropsy to the extent that he became reasonably comfortable for a few days. Several times in the next few months, when the kidney function had almost dried up, a vicarious intercession by the bowels virtually snatched the sick man from his grave. But it could not continue indefinitely. No excretory organ can assume completely the function of another.

There is good reason to believe that in his last years Jackson suffered from *cor pulmonale* (pulmonary heart), a mechanistic type of cardiac ailment arising from increased "back pressure" against the right half of the heart as it labors to force its contents through vessels constricted by pulmonary disease. The first result is hypertrophy, which in severe cases is followed by overstretching of muscle fibers and eventually by decompensation, dropsy, and death. In May, 1845, the General wrote a nephew, ". . . I am swollen from my toes to the crown of my head and in bandages to my hips." He was in the final phase of the last stage of right-sided heart failure. On June 2, Dr. Esselman of Nashville tapped the distended abdomen and obtained "much water" without giving appreciable relief. Opiates were freely administered, but the patient would not sleep. He talked of personal and national affairs with perfect lucidity. So it went to the morning of the last day, his body so far gone and his mind yet so clear as to suggest intelligence without corporeal dependence.

In his final hours, this son of America, who knew that the first stern requisites for a nation that would be great are room and resources, could view his country's prospects with profoundest satisfaction. He had wrested a vast territory from the aboriginal inhabitants, he had played a heavy role in the annexation of Florida, and he had persuaded Sam Houston to bring Texas into the Union. On June 6 he had written a letter to President Polk commending his stand on the Oregon question and expressing confidence of a settlement, peaceful or otherwise, to the advantage of the United States.

On June 8, 1845, his mission having been accomplished, the tired old soldier beckoned his friend, Death, who came and gently led him away into the darkness.

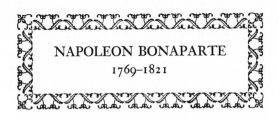

THE STORY OF NAPOLEON is essentially the story of a vast empire founded by the genius of one man and completely dependent upon him and his fortunes for its existence. For a time all went well. Then, though the founder was only a little more than forty years of age, insidious changes in personality, unrecognized at the time, began to assert themselves. Errors of judgment begetting dangerous situations were met with faltering action, and the inevitable penalties of indecision were blamed on the resistless force of Destiny. Collapse of the structure of empire, so precariously built and upheld, was swift and complete.

Medical scrutiny of his career strongly supports the thesis that the failures and the premature death of the great Bonaparte were respectively the trail marks and the terminus of a fairly common physical ailment, now largely subjugated by the achievements of medical science.

The biography of the famous soldier properly begins before his birth, for while yet in his mother's womb, he was repeatedly subjected to the hazards of battle. His mother, Letizia Buonaparte, had followed her husband to the war for independence which the Corsicans were waging against the French in 1769. "Often," said she, "in search of news I would steal from our mountain nook to the battlefield. I heard the bullets whistling but I put my trust in Our Lady." Following final defeat of the Islanders, Letizia's husband, Count Charles Buonaparte of Ajaccio, with other deputies, formally surrendered the island of Corsica to the French army. One month later, on August 15, the son, Napolione, was born. The conquerors dealt leniently with the nobility and, after a nine-year period of probation, King Louis made a grant of 2,000 francs to the Count and an award of a scholarship in the Nobles' School to each of the two older sons. One son was to become a priest; the other, an army officer. The latter, who was sent to the military school at Brienne, France, was Napoleon.

He was an undersized, poorly nourished boy, this Napolione, as he called himself, but impulsive and combative and, as a Corsican, resentful of his country's defeat and conquest by the French. Rated one of the school's best pupils, he was placed at the head of a company of boy cadets, but his "troops" held a council and denounced him as "unfit to command" because of his "lack of respect for his comrades." The sentence was demotion to the ranks and deprivation of insignia in the presence of his fellow cadets. He submitted to the degradation in a most soldierly manner, evincing no sense of either resentment or humiliation. His conduct on the trying occasion won for him a complete reversal of attitude on the part of the majority of his comrades. Here was a fellow who "could take it." They dubbed him "The Spartan." Action begot reaction, and he became a comparatively cheerful and friendly little chap except in the presence of those whom he regarded as "aristocratic snobs," a category in which he placed all who spoke disparagingly of Corsica or its people. Although his appearance was far from prepossessing and he had no athletic ability, yet he was somehow able to exact obedience from all in his group. He was the leader in mock warfare, especially in the designing and construction of ramparts and fortresses. It was evident that he had the innate gift of leadership.

His health at this time was only fair. He suffered frequent intestinal upsets, apparently of nervous origin, and he was allergic to cow's milk and dairy products. In 1784 he entered the military school at Paris, and after one year he was graduated a sub-lieutenant of artillery. His instructors made this final notation after his name: "Reserved and diligent, he prefers study to any kind of conversation and nourishes his mind upon good authors. He is taciturn with a love for solitude and is moody, overbearing, and extremely egotistical."

While at the Paris school he became embroiled with a priest to whom he had gone for confession. The father, after ascertaining the lad's nationality, denounced the Corsicans for a wicked lot, "insolent . . . bandits." Napoleon leaped to his feet, smashed the grille that separated them, and attacked the priest, who fought back furiously. Apparently little physical damage was done, but it is fair to believe that the tempestuous little Corsican departed from the church with less religion than he brought to it.

Upon graduation, the sixteen-year-old sub-lieutenant was given a new uniform, but he was so impecunious that he had to walk much of the way to Valence to join the regiment to which he was assigned. Shortly, his father died of cancer of the stomach, and Napoleon returned to Corsica on furlough. He spent a year with his own people, but it did not afford him the satisfaction he had expected. His family was without money, and the Corsican people seemed to have lost the fierce spirit of independence which once animated them. He wrote: "What a tragedy in the homeland! My fellowcountrymen, in chains, kiss the hand that beats them." With the expiration of his furlough, he returned to France. His orders directed him to proceed to a new post, Auxonne, a garrison town in the Côte-d'Or on the Saône River. The country was in turmoil; mobs were rioting and looting everywhere. Since he hated mobs as much as he hated the nobility, it was without compunction that he ordered his battery to fire on the rabble in the streets of Auxonne. Always, his thoughts turned to the homeland. Now that France was seething with internal strife, the time seemed opportune for Corsica to proclaim its freedom. He relished the thought that the King had spent money teaching him how to beat France and liberate Corsica. Under the law he was a complete traitor, but a Corsican could owe allegiance only to the country of his nativity. He applied for leave and it was granted.

As soon as he set foot on the homeland, he gathered his lieutenants and undertook to foment a rebellion against French rule. But the people were not ready to wager their lives and fortunes on the leadership of an inexperienced stripling, and the regular troops could not be intimidated. The cherished revolution died a-borning. The government wisely refrained from attempts to punish the conspirators, and the youthful patriot gained neither freedom for his people nor martyrdom for himself. He won a minor diplomatic success, however, by sponsoring an appeal to the newly created National Assembly in Paris which, in reply, granted the island provincial status with all the rights of other provinces under French dominion. He was not to be appeased; he would be satisfied with nothing less than absolute independence. He would try again and yet again. Meantime his last extension of leave had terminated, so he packed up and returned to his first post, the town of Valence.

The smoke of revolution was in the air of France. Louis XVI had made an ill-advised attempt to flee the country and was intercepted at Varennes. Finally came word that the virus of revolt had infected Corsica. Again Napoleon sought and obtained leave to return home. There was more work than could be done in the allotted time. He overstayed his leave and was cashiered from the French Army. On Easter Sunday, 1792, he led a sally by the citizens of Ajaccio against the fortress of the town. The attack failed miserably. A complaint charging armed rebellion was lodged against him in Paris and a trial for high treason was in prospect. Undaunted, he returned to the French capital and watched the storming of the Tuileries.

The new government not only took the deserter-traitor back into the service but also awarded him the rank of captain. He saw no reason, however, to concern himself with the troubles of France. So, instead of reporting to his regiment, he returned to his beloved Corsica. The island was in a state of virtual anarchy. By a political coup he was able to depose the conservative but nonetheless patriotic old Paoli and place himself, a captain in the French Army, in the position of commander. When an order came through from Paris for the arrest of Paoli, however, the people rallied to the defense of the honest old patriot, and, for the first time in his career, the brash young captain found himself fighting against his fellow Corsicans. The Buonaparte mansion was raided, and only by the grace of French protection was the family, including Napoleon, able to escape to a ship bound for Toulon. For a time he wandered about the country while the English, at the invitation of the well-to-do citizens of Toulon, occupied the tongue of land which extends into the bay in front of the city and divides the bay into two parts.

The problem of how to drive out the English interlopers confronted the commander of the port. A chance meeting with the idle captain of artillery solved the problem in brilliant fashion. Napoleon was wounded in the calf by an English lance, but the victory he achieved at Toulon was well worth the hazard and the pain. Two years after fleeing Ajaccio he was a brigadier-general in the French Army, and in two more he was commander of the army in Italy. The Revolution had been won, the war for Europe was underway, and the name of Napoleon was to be spoken in tones which will resound forever down the corridors of history.

It is difficult for us to realize, however well we may know it, that the body of a great genius is subject to the same ailments and his character to the same foibles as those affecting common mortals. As with many another, so with Napoleon, a knowledge of his personal life brings him down to earth with a somewhat sickening thud. But, of course, only the very naïve really expect the great to be also the good. Napoleon, for all his great physical and nervous endurance, never knew the joys of robust health. In 1789, while stationed at Auxonne, he developed a chronic fever, probably malaria, and was in ill health for many months. Nevertheless he worked with the persistence of a madman. At this time his appetite, never keen, failed him entirely. Frequently he would eat only a crust of bread during an entire day. It was his conviction that the less he ate the better he felt, which could well have been true in one of his enfeebled digestion. He often said that no matter how little a man eats, he eats too much. There can be no doubt but that during his late childhood and throughout the years of his adolescence he suffered not only from infectious disease but also from starvation, including a severe vitamin deficiency. There is reason to believe that at some time in his early life he had active pulmonary tuberculosis. Antommarchi, who conducted the autopsy at St. Helena, reported pleuritic adhesions on the left side as well as tubercles and numerous small tuberculous cavities in the upper lobe of the left lung.

"Civilization," said Talleyrand, "was always a little hateful to Napoleon." He considered the social amenities sheer nonsense—

155

frequently bathed in the presence of his servants or troops and ate with his fingers when usage demanded a spoon or fork. He took his food as if he were taking medicine. Apparently he ate strictly to live and got no enjoyment from his meals. Often he would jump from the table and hurry to his work masticating the last bite of food on the way. Sometimes he had no more than left the table when he was seized by an attack of severe abdominal pain which caused him to roll on the ground or floor cursing and moaning. These paroxysms of pain lasted only a few minutes and, because of their brief duration and their relation to meals, were probably due to nervous indigestion. Later in life he had attacks of what he called "stomach cramps," which were different from those just described and of much more serious import.

During the Italian campaign he was tortured by the itch (scabies), an affection which any housewife today can cure with sulfur and lard but which was a complete puzzle to the doctors of Napoleon's time. He cursed and reviled his physicians, who dosed him with potions and plastered him with ointments all to no benefit. Meantime he had communicated the disease to his wife, Josephine, who, it is safe to suppose, supplied whatever was lacking to fill the cup of his misery. Finally, he called in the famous doctor Corvisart who knew how to cure the disease even if he did not know its cause. Corvisart prescribed a mixture of alcohol, olive oil, and powdered cevadilla for external use. The last-named substance contains the drug, veratrine, which has been used effectively against pediculosis (lousiness) and probably therefore would also cure the itch, which is caused by a tiny parasite, the *acarus scabiei*.

At about the age of thirty, Napoleon began to suffer from cystitis which manifested itself in the form of frequent, painful urination. Sometimes he was observed to rest his head against a tree or wall and moan with pain as he passed his water. The cause of his cystitis was revealed at his autopsy when numerous small stones were found in his bladder. He was also found to have gallstones and it is very likely that some of his severest attacks of abdominal pain were, in fact, gallstone colic.

A final answer to the question whether Napoleon was or was not epileptic will probably never be forthcoming. It has been definitely established, however, that he did on several occasions suffer some sort of fit in which his face became distorted, he appeared to lose consciousness, and he fell to the ground. Sometimes vomiting followed the seizure. But he did not chew his tongue nor lose control of bladder or bowels, and he regained consciousness quickly without relapsing into stupor. The seizures as described, were too severe for Petit Mal and too mild for Grand Mal. In modern times, correlation of "brain waves" registered by the encephalograph, with visible symptoms exhibited by patients has broadened the scope of the term "epilepsy" to include "attacks" whose relationship to the disease was heretofore unsuspected. In the light of our newer knowledge, it would seem that Napoleon had an atypical epilepsy. If, as has been stated, one or two seizures occurred during sleep, that fact would lend clinical weight to the diagnosis. The seizures were by no means habitual. Only four or five are recorded. Talleyrand tells of witnessing a convulsive fit at Strasbourg, and the Emperor's *valet de chambre*, Constant, has described three similar paroxysms. Another occurred under highly embarrassing circumstances when one of his mistresses, the actress Mlle Georg, was spending the night with him. Discovering the Emperor in convulsions by her side, she sprang from the bed shrieking in terror. The whole household came running to the room. Suddenly Napoleon "came to" and seeing his wife, Josephine, and all the servants gathered around his bed, flew into a terrible rage. He ordered everyone to get out of the room instantly and the next day he commanded Mlle Georg to leave Paris. The episode marked the end of their intimacy.

In general, Napoleon held physicians in contempt, though he placed a high value on surgeons, who were, as a group, active and courageous men of his own type. Surgeons could see what they were about: they could save lives and they were useful in improving or maintaining the morale of the army. Of his chief surgeon he wrote, "Larrey is the most virtuous man I have ever known." And again, "He was the most honest man and the best friend of the soldiers that I have ever met. Vigilant and indefatigable, one could find Larrey with the wounded at all hours of the day or night trying to discern some sign of life in the bodies stretched on the ground." Apparently, the one physician for whom he felt any deep respect or admiration was Corvisart, the doctor who cured him of itch.

With respect to women, he always cherished a chivalrous and tender regard for the sweethearts of his innocent youth. Désirée Eugénie Clary, to whom he once proposed marriage, which was refused, wrote him a heart-broken letter following his marriage to Josephine de Beauharnais. Later Désirée was married to General Bernadotte, a Jacobin, a hater of Napoleon, and a thorough hypocrite. In order to benefit Désirée, Napoleon made Bernadotte marshal of the Empire and Knight of the Black Eagle. Caught in a conspiracy against the First Consul (Napoleon), Bernadotte escaped punishment purely on account of Désirée. The Consul's lenity soon cost him dearly, for Bernadotte was to play a villain's role in the drama of the last days of the Empire. With women whose company he sought for mere gratification, Napoleon was brutal and contemptuous. Toward cultured, attractive women, he was inclined to be excessively idealistic. Sometimes, apparently, he avoided further association with some woman he had idealized lest a perfectionistic concept be shattered. It would seem that he knowingly indulged in illusions.

It was a harsh decree of Fate that Napoleon should be wed to a woman whom he loved to distraction but who, in her turn, was openly unfaithful and unappreciative of his devotion. When eventually he expressed dissatisfaction with their sterile union, hinting at divorce, Josephine became jealous and went into hysterical fits of weeping. It was not that she had a sudden love for her husband; she was thinking only of herself and her position. Believing that her marriage could be saved if she could have a child—in fact, Napoleon had said as much—she visited spas, physicians, quacks, and soothsayers. Several times, deceived by her menstrual irregularity, both she and her husband thought she was pregnant, but every hope failed of realization. In 1804, Napoleon was proclaimed emperor and a son became a necessity, but he waited six years more to divorce Josephine and take in her stead Marie Louise, the stupid, seventeen-year-old daughter of the Emperor of Austria. His one true love was the Polish Countess Walewski who came to him in terror, a pawn for her country, but remained to love him as no other woman ever did. She gave him everything a woman can give a man, asked nothing for herself, and in his days of defeat, displayed the same tender devotion as in the days of his glory.

He had three sons and no daughters. His one legitimate heir was by Marie Louise; of the two illegitimates, one, Léon, was the child of a nameless woman to whom Napoleon was introduced by his sister, Carolina, and the other, Alexander, was a son of Countess Walewski. The legitimate heir, Napoleon II, died of pulmonary tuberculosis at the age of twenty-one; Léon came to America, married a cook, and died obscurely; while Alexander, as Count Walewski, won distinction as minister of state and senator in the Second Empire.

Bonaparte considered sleep an unfortunate necessity and preferred frequent short naps to a solid night's slumber. He was able to go to sleep whenever he felt the need for it, and he could awaken at any hour previously fixed in his mind. During battle, if affairs seemed to be going well, he could doze in the saddle even in situations of personal danger. He was an avid reader and carried a library, sometimes of several hundred volumes, with him on his campaigns. In a factual world, he could see no sense in fiction though he enjoyed poetry and fairy tales. Science and mathematics occupied most of his attention. He read and conversed in Italian, French, and English with almost equal fluency and had considerably more than a smattering of German and Spanish. His Italian accent was more noticeable in his French than in his English. Personally, he rarely did any writing, and when he wrote his spelling was bad, his sentences often unfinished, and his script undecipherable. He was the despair of his secretaries, whom he worked unmercifully. "I know just how far my feet can carry me and I know the limits of my sight," he once said, "but I have never discovered the limits of my capacity for work. I can easily kill six secretaries." He would sometimes keep four secretaries busy simultaneously as he dictated on a different subject to each. Despite the great rapidity of dictation, his thought was clear and his phraseology superb. The tempo of his intellectual processes was phenomenally fast; his muscular movements were relatively slow.

When work was to be done, he was in a constant state of impatience. If riding in a carriage, he was continually shouting at the coachman to drive "faster, faster!" He was not a skilled horseman, but he usually rode his mount at a gallop. Nothing else roused his anger so much as unnecessary delay. Once his mind had settled on a course of action, he wished to start forthwith. He desired to encourage the growth of Paris and asked his minister of the interior for suggestions. "The City needs much good water: the water supply is bad," said the Minister, who then sketched a plan for diverting the Orcq to the capital by means of a canal. Napoleon studied the sketch and asked questions. Then with finality he said, "The project is sound; send 500 men to LaVilet tomorrow to start the canal."

His memory was extraordinary. Every fact that fell within its scope seemed permanently fixed. "I know not only all the officers' names in every regiment of France," he once declared, "but also the regions from which these troops were drafted, at what engagements they distinguished themselves, and their political inclinations."

During the years of the Consulate, he was a beneficent leader and ruler; his sense of service motivating every act. "It is my policy," he said, "to govern men as the majority of them wish to be governed. This, I believe, is the best way of recognizing the sovereignty of the people." As he grew older, however, he wished not so much to serve as to be served. He maintained that the final objective of his campaigns, military and civil, was the creation of a United States of Europe. "We need a European legal code, a European court of appeal, a unified coinage, a common system of weights and measures. The same law must run throughout Europe. I shall fuse all nations into one." Such was the fair flower which was to spring from the blood-soaked soil of Europe. His craving for power was insatiable. "Yes," he admitted in the days of his misfortune, "I desire to rule the world. Who would not have desired it had he been in my place?"

With increased power and declining health, his natural irascibility became more and more evident. Once, when Dr. Corvisart made his daily call at the Tuileries to inquire after the Emperor's health, he found him in a maniacal fury, terrorizing everyone about the place. It was with great difficulty that the doctor was able to elicit the cause of the imperial rage—a splinter of toothpick stuck between two of the Emperor's teeth. After Corvisart had removed the offending particle, the great man regained his composure at once and proceeded with his work as if nothing had happened. In moments of great agitation his mouth twitched and his left calf trembled violently, phenomena distantly related to the seizures of epilepsy. He was naturally destructive even in a state of calmness. It is told that he rarely entered the greenhouses at Fontainebleau without breaking stems or leaves of some of the rare tropical plants sheltered there.

In his softer moments he was easily touched and even roused to tears. Once when leaving for a campaign he wept so violently as he bade Josephine and Talleyrand adieu that he became sick and vomited. He wept at the deathbed of the faithful general, Massena, and he is said to have cried before the Battle of Waterloo. He greatly admired bravery and candor. When the German youth, Staps, forced his way into the palace at Schönbrunn for the purpose of assassinating the Emperor, the intended victim would not consent to have the brave fellow shot until the youth had assured him that if pardoned he would surely try again. On another occasion, following a tirade against physicians and their ethics, Napoleon was astounded to receive a signed letter from an obscure army doctor named Pugnet. The letter read: "You are a conqueror—that is to say, you are one who sacrifices everything for your own interest, your own glory. Remain a conqueror, pursue your career of destruction, but respect those who, having no other goal than the welfare of humanity, give their lives to repair the evils caused by you and your like." He summoned the young physician, took him gently by the ear and said: "Doctor Pugnet, you come from the South; you have a hot head but an excellent heart. Some day, in spite of your pride, you will come to ask a favor and I shall be glad to grant it." Pugnet did not delay the request. He replied that he would like nothing better than to be transferred to Martinique to study yellow fever. Napoleon was delighted. "You," said he, "are a real doctor." The transfer was arranged at once.

As he approached the age of forty, Napoleon began to grow fat and sluggish. During the Russian campaign in 1812, he suffered from swelling of the legs and he manifested an indecision quite unlike the Napoleon of previous campaigns. At Dresden the follow-

Medical Biographies

ing year he maneuvered brilliantly but because of a "gastric attack," he was unable to follow through and clinch the victory. Just before Leipzig he suffered another "gastric attack" and during the retreat of his army was so badly exhausted that he fell into a deep sleep while his generals waited around the fire for their chief to wake up. Plainly he was no longer the "man of iron" or the magician of the battlefield. He was just a sick man. Many of his oldest and most trusted officers, losing faith in both his intentions and his fitness to command, deserted and even went over to the enemy. The crash could not be averted—the allies entered Paris, the Emperor was forced to abdicate, and then almost exactly one year after Lützen he sailed under guard for Elba.

During his ten months at Elba, he built a toy kingdom and played a mixed role of country squire, warrior, and emperor. He seemed to be enjoying one of the remissions characteristic of the chronic disease from which he suffered. Upon his return to France he displayed a verve and energy reminiscent of his better days, but when he got to Paris, it was noted that he was fat, his features sagged, his complexion was sallow, and he dozed or slept with an unprecedented disregard for the vast amount of work confronting him. His plans for the Battle of Waterloo, however, were worthy of his former genius, but he faltered in their execution. The result is known to all. Rout of his army by the allies and his personal surrender to the English made Waterloo a lasting byword for complete and final defeat.

As the *Bellerophon* bore him toward Plymouth, Napoleon felt himself fortunate to be a captive guest of the English, but he soon found to his dismay that he had reckoned without his host. When confronted with the government decree condemning him to imprisonment on St. Helena, he refused to sign, reminding the British that he had given himself up voluntarily when avenues of escape were open and that, contrary to the assertions of the document, St. Helena was a pest-ridden spot which would kill him in three months. With his physician, O'Meara, three officers, and twelve servants, he was transferred to the *Northumberland* which shortly set sail for St. Helena. As he reflected upon the perfidy and inhumanity of official England, his resentment must have cooled a little at recollection of the common folk who, with uncovered heads, crowded the port of Plymouth to get a glimpse of the "caged monster" and to pay honest respect to the most stupendous personality of the age.

St. Helena is a mass of volcanic rock, forty-seven square miles in area, projecting from the waters of the South Atlantic at a point approximately one thousand miles from the equator and about the same distance from the coast of Africa. Originally the island was so sterile that it was necessary to import hundreds of shiploads of humus in order that officers and families stationed there by the East India Company and the British government might grow necessary garden vegetables. The climate is similar to that prevailing on small islands of the Caribbean in northern equatorial waters. In the time of Napoleon the total population was about 1,700 of whom 1,200 were Negroes or Chinese, most of whom undoubtedly carried the *entamoeba histolytica*, the causal organism of amoebic dysentery, in their intestinal tracts. In regions where amoebic dysentery is endemic will be found many carriers, persons who harbor the organism and show no symptoms of the disease but are capable of communicating the malady to uninfected persons. Once the mucous membrane of the colon is invaded, however, the characteristic diarrhoea appears, followed in severe cases by fever and, not uncommonly, by liver abscess and death. When Dr. O'Meara, Napoleon's physician wrote, "The most prevalent complaints are dysentery, inflammation of the bowels, liver affections and fevers —all of them generally violent in form," he was unaware that he was, for the most part, talking about a single disease. But when he further observed that "the dysentery and liver affections are frequently combined," he must have suspected a common cause. The "liver affections" mentioned by O'Meara were commonly called "hepatitis" by the physicians of the time and designated with inflammatory process in the liver, including abscesses of amoebic origin.

The *Northumberland* put in at Jamestown, St. Helena, on October 17, 1815. At first the deposed Emperor lived in the quiet Valley of the Briars, but after two months he was moved to Longwood on the barren, wind-swept southern slope of the island. Here he and his retinue lived in quarters made out of a cowshed, a washhouse, and a stable. The place was damp, mouldy, and overrun by rats. His custody and general care were in the hands of Sir Hudson Lowe, former chief of espionage in Italy and now governor of St. Helena. The life of Sir Hudson seemed dominated by two emotions, an insane fear that his prisoner might escape and an egoistic pleasure in ruling the man who had once ruled most of Europe. After Lowe's first visit, the Emperor exclaimed, "Execrable! A real hang-dog face, like that of a Venetian sbirro. . . . Perhaps he is my executioner."

While the Governor was giving lavish dinners, Napoleon was allowed only the poorest fare. He could not get even fresh water. Nevertheless, his health was moderately good during the first year; the second year he developed scurvy, which was relieved by the addition of lime juice to his diet. In the spring of 1817 he suffered a recurrence of the swelling of his legs, a condition which had bothered him periodically since the Russian campaign. The swelling was of the orthostatic type, which is to say it came after he had been on his feet for a while and gradually disappeared after he lay down. His stomach trouble grew worse, and for the first time he complained of pain below the ribs on the right side. Doctor O'-Meara noted that "the right side felt firmer to pressure than the left" and there was some pain response to "hard pressure." Further, "His legs still swollen, especially towards night . . . and symptoms of dyspepsia such as nausea and flatulence." Meantime the fact of the Emperor's poor health had been bruited about, and the moderates in England joined the French in protesting the treatment accorded the prisoner. Governor Lowe reacted to the criticism in a manner worthy of the petty tyrant he was by imposing even more severe restrictions.

The French set up the cry that the Emperor had hepatitis due to the unhealthful climate of St. Helena. Dr. O'Meara, who had already won the Governor's enmity by refusing to act the spy for him, concurred in the diagnosis of hepatitis and was recalled to England to receive a strong official rebuke. Before leaving the island, however, the physician, in direct disobedience of orders, made a furtive visit to take an affectionate leave of his patient. As Napoleon had refused to see Dr. Baxter, whom the Governor had chosen to take O'Meara's post, he had no physician at all the next year. Consequently no medical records were kept. Madame Ber-

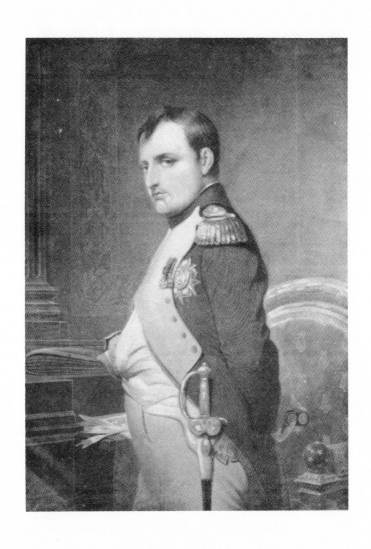

NAPOLEON BONAPARTE

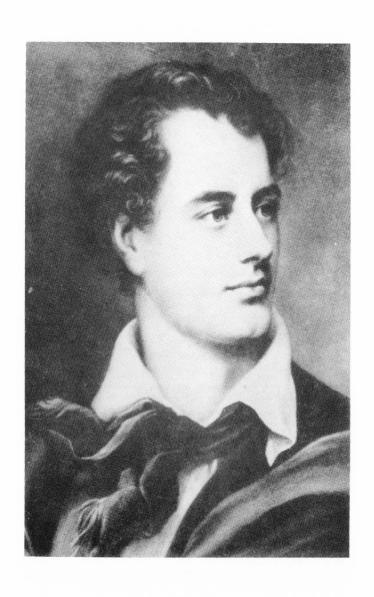

LORD BYRON

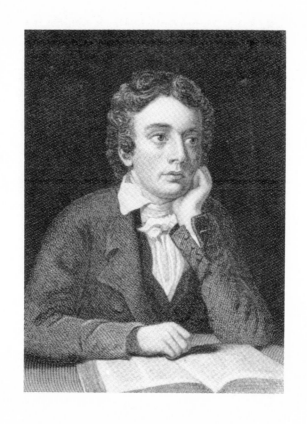

JOHN KEATS

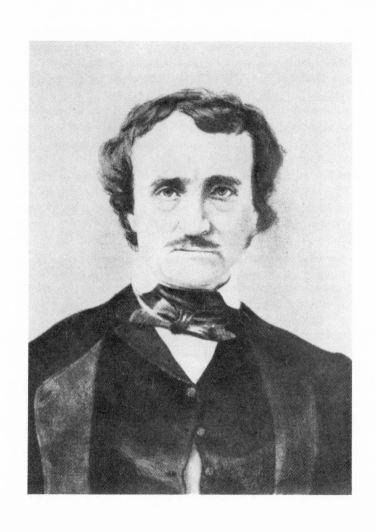

EDGAR ALLAN POE

trand, wife of one of the three French officers permitted to accompany the Emperor, tells us, however, that he continued to suffer periods of bad health when "his eyes were tired, his complexion yellowish and leaden, pointing to a chronic disease."

On January 16, 1819, the Emperor had an attack resembling apoplexy, which again brought up the problem of medical care. Dr. John Stokoe, inspector of naval hospitals, was brought in. Stokoe visited the sick man several times and in the end was courtmartialed for "making a thoughtless, incautious diagnosis of the patient's disease and of addressing him with a title expressly prohibited by act of Parliament." Stokoe had reported that the Emperor was extremely weak and suffered "from a great pain on the right side in the hepatic region." The physician also wrote to General Bertrand, "It appears from the symptoms that chronic hepatitis is the principal cause of the patient's poor health. I do not believe there is any immediate danger, but hepatitis is a dangerous disease, particularly in a climate like that of St. Helena." Stokoe was forced to resign from the navy, and again Napoleon was without a physician. The prisoner was now chronically ailing. His legs swelled whenever he was on his feet for a little while, his complexion was sallow, his hearing and sight failing, and he spent most of the day either in bed or in a hot bath. Once, surprisingly enough, he suddenly became more energetic and cheerful. It was evident that his ailment was one characterized by relapses and remissions. He was in fair health for almost a year, but Dr. Antommarchi, a fellow Corsican who had been hired by the Emperor's mother and had arrived meantime, still found symptoms of liver disease.

In mid-July, 1820, the Emperor had an acute relapse marked by fever, headache, and vomiting of bile. From then on he suffered increasingly frequent attacks of pain in the gall-bladder region, diarrhoea, and cough, the symptoms appearing either singly or together. The end of the year found him extremely weak and pale. Antommarchi insisted on dosing the patient against all reason. Napoleon hated the physician, whose ignorant insistence that he try this or that drug had caused him much nausea and discomfort. Governor Lowe expressed the opinion that the prisoner was suffering from "a slight anemia" and would soon recover. Antommarchi theorized that the trouble was "remittent gastric fever." Dr. Archibald Arnott was called by Lowe as consultant. Arnott reported that because of the darkness of the room in which the patient was confined, "I was unable to see him at all. But I could feel him or someone else." The pulse and the state of the pain pointed to considerable disability but there was nothing that indicated immediate danger.

The following day Arnott again visited the sick man and made an examination. "Sire," said Arnott, "it is not your liver that is affected. You have inflammation of the stomach." Napoleon seemed both surprised and alarmed. "But," said he, "I have always had an excellent stomach. Yet, recently I began to feel a sharp, piercing pain that cut into me like a razor. My father died of stomach trouble at the age of thirty-eight. Is it hereditary?" Arnott replied that the type of pain described by the Emperor was consistent with ulceration of the stomach, but he was convinced that it was mere inflammation. Despite the patient's increasing weakness and loss of weight, Arnott maintained officially that the trouble was of neurotic origin. Napoleon, convinced that he was going to die soon, made his will and also dictated a letter to Montholon which was to be delivered to Governor Lowe immediately upon the advent of death. The letter read: "Your Excellency: The Emperor died on [date] as a result of a long and painful illness. I have the honor to inform you of that fact. Please let me know what arrangements your government has made for conveyance of his body to Europe and also in respect of the members of his suite."

The accelerated deterioration in the prisoner's condition could no longer be denied, and Governor Lowe, who had pooh-poohed the suggestion of danger, now became alarmed. He had been reporting to the British War Office that the patient's illness was mere hysteria. Demise at this time would be exceedingly embarrassing not only to the Governor but also to official England, which had been bitterly assailed at home and abroad for inconsiderate or even brutal treatment of the celebrated prisoner. Lowe called for a medical consultation. Three English physicians, Drs. Arnott, Shortt, and Mitchell, together with the Corsican Antommarchi, met in a room at Longwood by request of the Governor. After a brief discussion it was decided that it would be advantageous to see the patient himself—a reasonable conclusion. But Napoleon refused them. So they played Hamlet with Hamlet *in absentia*. It was their considered opinion that the patient's condition demanded a large dose of calomel. As the Emperor had already had a surfeit of inspirational medication, he refused to co-operate. Probably as a matter of policy rather than a matter of wisdom, Antommarchi opposed the recommendation of the English doctors. But the latter approached Marchand, who, being persuaded that only a dose of calomel could stay the hand of death, concealed the drug in sweetened water and gave it to the sick man. Napoleon swallowed the mixture and then turned reproachfully to Marchand, "You too, deceived me?"—a rebuke which was to ring in the ears of Marchand as long as he lived. Almost immediately the Emperor went into a state of collapse, from which, after about thirty minutes, he revived violently to spring from his bed in delirium and throttle Montholon, who was alone with him, in a vise-like grip. In a moment his hands relaxed and he sank to the floor. He was then placed back in bed, where he lay breathing quietly. The stupor deepened and finally, a few minutes before six o'clock on the evening of May 5, 1821, all bodily functions ceased.

The following morning Governor Lowe viewed the corpse and ordered an immediate autopsy. Antommarchi reminded him that the law required an interval of twenty-four hours between the instant of death and the commencement of post-mortem section. Turning to his assistant, Admiral Reade, the Governor ordered him to be present at the autopsy, which would take place at two o'clock in the afternoon. At the appointed time, Antommarchi, enormously pleased with his role of autopsy surgeon, undertook the dissection in the presence of five English army surgeons, three English army officers, and three Frenchmen.

It was noted that the body was uniformly covered by a substantial layer of fat. There was much discussion and some argument at each step of the dissection. Three reports of the findings were made, the official one signed by all the British doctors except Henry, a semi-official one by Dr. Henry in 1823, and another by Antommarchi on behalf of himself and the French representatives. The report of Antommarchi disagreed with the first in some important details. The official report states:

167

A trifling adhesion of the left pleura to the pleura costalis was found; about 3 oz. of reddish fluid were contained in the left cavity and nearly 8 oz. in the right. The lungs were quite sound. The pericardium was natural and contained about an ounce of fluid. The heart was of the natural size but thickly covered with fat. The auricles and ventricles exhibited nothing extraordinary except that the muscular parts appeared rather paler than natural. Upon opening the abdomen the omentum was found remarkably fat and, on exposing the stomach that viscus was found the seat of extensive disease; strong adhesions connected the whole superior surface, particularly about the pyloric extremity, to the concave surface of the liver; and on separating these an ulcer which penetrated the coats of the stomach was discovered one inch from the pylorus, sufficient to allow passage of the little finger. The internal surface of the stomach to nearly its whole extent was a mass of cancerous disease or scirrhous portions advancing to cancer: this was particularly noticed near the pylorus. The cardiac extremity for a small space near the termination of the oesophagus was the only part appearing in a healthy state. The stomach was found nearly filled with a large quantity of fluid resembling coffee grounds.[1] The convex surface of the left lobe of the liver adhered to the diaphragm but with the exception of the adhesions occasioned by disease in the stomach no unhealthy appearance presented itself in the liver. The remainder of the abdominal viscera were in a healthy state. A slight peculiarity in the shape of the left kidney was observed.

(Signed) Shortt, Arnott, Burton,
Livingstone, Mitchell.

The heart and stomach were placed in separate containers which were filled with spirits and sealed hermetically.

Dr. Henry, it appears, capriciously refused to sign the report. Antommarchi, as stated elsewhere, reported tubercles and numerous small tuberculous cavities in the upper lobe of the left lung. The organs were not weighed or measured as would be done to-

[1] Blood which has undergone granular clotting.

day and, of course, no tissue was removed for microscopic study as that science was still unknown.

Several of the post-mortem findings deserve comment:

In 1925 the eminent British surgeon and pathologist, Sir Berkeley Moynihan, stated: "I have had the opportunity of examining the viscera of Napoleon and found there absolutely no trace of cancer." Moreover, there could scarcely have been a stomach cancer of the severity and duration indicated in the official report without invasion of the liver to such an extent that gross changes could not be overlooked. In the absence of such changes and in view of Lord Moynihan's statement there is good reason to doubt that the ulcer had become cancerous at all. Certainly the Emperor did not die of cancer of the stomach as is commonly asserted. His *demise resulted from perforated peptic ulcer, hemorrhage, and peritonitis.* Since the science of pathology was in its infancy in their time, the autopsy surgeons are not to be censured for their failure to distinguish between cancer and inflammatory changes adjacent to the ulcerated area.

Although the official report declares that "the lungs were quite sound," Antommarchi claims to have observed and called to the attention of the others "numerous tubercles and small cavities" involving the upper lobe of the left lung. Antommarchi's assertion receives some clinical support in the history of a prolonged period of ill health of unknown cause while Napoleon was stationed at Valence, a persistent cough during the Italian campaign, a "walking illness" with expectoration of blood in 1803, and, finally, the death of his son, Napoleon II, of pulmonary tuberculosis at the age of twenty-one.

When it is recalled that during the Russian campaign in 1812 the Emperor first developed swelling of the legs in association with weakness, sallow complexion, and loss of incentive and that the symptom complex disappeared and recurred at intervals throughout the rest of his life, we must conclude that severe periodic anemia due to slow but prolonged leakages of blood from his chronic peptic ulcer was the chief cause of the fluctuations in the state of his health.

Clinical experience has shown that in almost every instance of chronic deeply penetrating gastric or duodenal ulcer some degree of intermittent hemorrhage occurs. If the resultant anemia is severe and the patient is up and about, swelling of the lower extremities (orthostatic edema) commonly results from seepage of the thinned blood plasma through the walls of the capillaries. In dark-complexioned persons the skin becomes sallow or yellowish, in the light-complexioned it becomes ghastly pale. A frequent and often unnoted symptom is the passage of "tarry" stools. After weeks or months the bleeding may cease spontaneously and permit the victim to recover his appearance of health and his sense of well-being before another spell occurs. Always there are the lurking dangers of sudden severe hemorrhage, perforation with resulting peritonitis, and, in cases of gastric ulcer, malignant degenerative changes among the epithelial cells bordering on the crater of the ulcer.

Every case of deep-seated peptic ulcer requires medical care in the widest sense of the term. This implies the energetic employment of proper dietary, drug, and psychological measures always, with resort to surgery occasionally. Given the patient's full cooperation, great improvement may be expected in almost every instance with healing of the ulcer in more than 80 per cent of cases.

Nowadays Napoleon's ulcer could probably be cured, but to achieve that desideratum the Little Corporal would be compelled to shun the tensions of the battlefield.

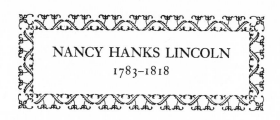

ALMOST NOTHING is recorded of the early life of Nancy Hanks Lincoln, mother of our sixteenth president, and much that has been told of her later life is fanciful and contradictory. It happens, however, that there has been preserved for us a fairly trustworthy account of the manner of her death.

It seems possible that the circumstances related to Nancy's origin may have been purposely concealed. Beveridge cites evidence that she was of illegitimate birth, noting that "in Elizabethtown [Kentucky] there dwelt one Joseph Hanks, a carpenter by trade. . . . Joseph Hanks had a niece, Nancy, the natural child of his sister, Lucy Hanks, and this girl was destined to become the mother of Abraham Lincoln. For some years she had made her home with an aunt, Betsy Sparrow, who had been married to Thomas Sparrow." Beveridge further states that "the father of Nancy Hanks is unknown, although in an unwonted burst of confidence Lincoln told his law partner that his maternal grandfather was a 'well bred Virginia planter,' and from this source flowed, as Lincoln believed, his noblest powers."

No portrait of Nancy has been left us and descriptions of her appearance are conflicting. One man who in his youth lived in her neighborhood has depicted her as "short and heavy." The testimony of several others, however, indicates that in her mature years she was above average height and had rather a spare frame. Her hair was black or very dark and her eyes are believed to have been blue. Her cousin, Dennis Hanks, who as a lad probably saw more of her than did any of the neighbors, described her "as pretty as a picture and as smart as you'd find them anywhere. She could read and write." Almost certainly Dennis is mistaken in saying that she could write, for a deed executed on October 27, 1814, transferring ownership of the Lincoln farm in Hardin County, Kentucky, to Thomas Melton, was signed by Nancy with a wavering cross-mark. The name of Thomas Lincoln was apparently appended by his own hand. Illiterate as Nancy probably was, she was nevertheless endowed with much good sense and had a kind and affectionate nature. Abraham Lincoln, who was nine years of age at the time of her death, seems to have rarely made mention of his mother in later years and then only to praise her wisdom and motherly goodness.

After disposing of their Kentucky farm, the Lincoln family, consisting of the husband and father, Thomas Lincoln, Nancy, a daughter, Sarah, and little Abe, moved to Indiana. There in the dense woods along Pigeon Creek, so called because of the wild pigeons which swarmed over the region in "pigeon season," Thomas built a rude log structure which served as a house for the family. In the spring of 1817 he returned to Kentucky to fetch a cow and a few pigs to the new home in the wilderness. There was no open pasture for the cow, so she was belled and turned loose in the woods to find such forage as she might in a locality practically destitute of grass. In the autumn of 1817, Nancy's aunt and uncle, Betsy and Thomas Sparrow, crossed the Ohio to Indiana and took up their abode close to that of the Lincolns.

All went reasonably well until the fall of 1818 when an epidemic of what was called "milk sickness" struck the little community of Pigeon Creek. Some of the more observant settlers in the Ohio basin had previously noted that the sickness seemed to be associated with a disease of cattle called "trembles," and they astutely ascribed it to the consumption of dairy products from cows which had eaten some kind of poisonous herb. The characteristic symptoms in humans were a sense of fatigue, stiffness and weakness of the legs, and abdominal distress in the early stages, followed by vomiting and severe prostration. The tongue was red, the pulse weak, and the temperature subnormal. Although some of the stricken persons recovered after lingering on the brink of death for weeks, many died from two to nine days after the onset of symptoms. Bulger *et al.* assert without speculative qualification that in pioneer days milk sickness "caused appalling loss of human life."

In September, Thomas and Betsy Sparrow were stricken with the disease. The nearest doctor was thirty-five miles away, but even if he had been at hand, he could have done nothing to arrest the progress of the malady and very little to alleviate the suffering of its victims. Nancy nursed them as well as she was able, but the elderly couple succumbed within a few hours of each other. Thomas Lincoln fashioned a pair of rude coffins out of the trunks of freshly fallen trees, using pegs in lieu of nails, and the two bodies were buried side by side on a wooded hilltop near the makeshift cabin which had been their home. A neighbor woman, Mrs. Peter Brooner, was also down with the sickness and Nancy nursed her a few days until the poor woman died. Shortly after, Nancy herself fell a victim of the sickness and took to her rough bed of leaves and corn husks. Evidently she early realized that she could not survive, for on the fourth or fifth day she called Sarah and Abraham to her side, bade them be good children, and kissed them good-bye. She died October 5, 1818, on the seventh day of her illness. For her, as for each of the others, the rugged, patient, bumbling Thomas made a crude coffin. Her remains were laid beside those of her Aunt Betsy and Uncle Tom.

It took the scientists a long time to confirm the observation of the early settlers that milk sickness is due to the use of dairy products of animals that have eaten a poisonous plant. The decreasing incidence of the disease, whether viewed as trembles in cattle or milk sickness in humans, probably accounts for the dearth of scientific attention which has been accorded it. From time to time experiments had been made, notably by Moseley, Curtis, and Sackett, which indicated that white snakeroot, also called richweed (*Eupatorium urticaefolium*), was the offender, but it remained for James Fitton Couch not only to reproduce the disease in animals but to isolate and identify the toxic agent as well (1927). Couch named the poisonous principle *trematol* and stated that it exists partly in the free state and partly in ester combination with a resinous acid. It is commonly stated that the sickness may be acquired by eating the meat of affected animals, but Couch was unable to reproduce the symptoms in a cat which was fed the giblets of a rabbit killed by trematol poisoning.

White snakeroot is thus described in the language of botany: "A smooth or nearly smooth branching herb from two to three feet high, leaves opposite, thin, rounded, cordate at the base or abruptly narrowed into a slender petiole, coarsely and sharply toothed; heads in loose cymose clusters, flowers white, involucre campanulate, bracts linear, acute or acuminate." The area of distribution embraces both the Ohio and the Mississippi valleys. Animals permitted to run in dense woods are especially likely to be affected, but even so some woods are safe while others are dangerous.

Grazing animals will not eat white snakeroot unless forced to it by a lack of normal pasturage. It is said that in the first half of the nineteenth century many settlers who came to Ohio from Pennsylvania returned to the home state upon learning of the menace to their families and cattle. Thomas Lincoln, however, chose to move farther west, to Illinois, when some years after the death of Nancy Hanks a second epidemic of milk sickness struck the Pigeon Creek region. The Lincolns were spared further experience with the disease, though the wooded areas of Illinois were probably about as dangerous as those of Indiana. In the course of an epidemic of trembles in the vicinity of Minooka, Illinois, early in the present century, more than fifty head of cattle are reported to have died of the disease. Numerous instances of trembles and milk sickness are known to have occurred in the high range country of New Mexico and Arizona. There the disease is due to another herb, the "jimmey weed" or rayless goldenrod (*Aplopappus heterophyllus*), but the toxic substance is identical with that found in white snakeroot.

According to Couch, Thienes, and others, trematol is an aromatic, optically active, straw-colored oil occurring in white snakeroot and rayless goldenrod. When excreted in milk it is susceptible of chemical identification. Symptoms resulting from ingestion of the toxic substance are chiefly assignable to the extreme degree of acidosis which it induces. The breath has the characteristic odor of acetone and excessive amounts of acetone are present in the blood. In cattle and sheep, trembling is uniformly present, and this symptom is responsible for the name attached to the disease in animals. In fatal cases of milk sickness or trembles, extensive degenerative changes are found in the liver, kidney, pancreas, and other vital organs.

Although the treatment of milk sickness is wholly symptomatic, yet, if begun early, it is fairly effective. The importance of rest is emphasized by the observation that persons or animals harboring the toxin may show little or no evidence of illness so long as physical activity is avoided but may quickly succumb after moderate muscular exertion. If begun early, intravenous injections of alkalies and glucose in proper dosage can be depended upon to control acidosis and protect vital organs against destructive changes.

It is an interesting fact that the mountaineers of the Southwest compounded a medicine of their own for milk sickness. It consisted essentially of a mixture of brandy and honey. The best that can be said for the brandy is that it gave comfort; but the honey, by providing a highly concentrated and quickly assimilable carbohydrate, exerted a definitely antagonistic action upon the acidosis. It is quite possible that the severity of the symptoms was often reduced and the lives of affected persons sometimes saved through the use of this primitive remedy of purely impulsive origin.

With the advent of extensive cultivation of the soil, better care of livestock, and an aversion to the use of milk of ailing cows, instances of milk sickness have become extremely rare.

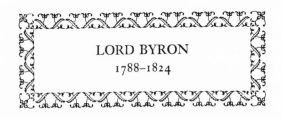

LORD BYRON
1788–1824

GEORGE GORDON NOEL BYRON, famous poet and infamous rake, was born on Holles Street, London, the son of "Mad Jack" Byron, officer of the Guards, and Catherine Gordon, Scottish heiress and vixen. It is recorded that the infant son came into the world wearing a caul,[1] which, according to the superstition of the times, marked him as one predestined to a long life and a happy one. The caul itself was preserved and sold to Mr. Hanson, the family solicitor, who gave it to his brother, Captain Hanson, R. N., as a charm against the perils of the sea. Apparently its prophylactic virtues were not very lasting, for two years later, off Newstead, the Captain's ship went down with all hands.

Lord Byron was lame from birth, but the exact nature of his disability has never been established. *The Dictionary of National Biography*, in common with several other biographical works, declares that the lameness affected both feet. That assertion is probably founded on a statement made in the writings of Edward John Trelawny, who, though he was a close friend and companion of Byron, was so habitually careless in his treatment of factual material that his word cannot be accepted as authoritative. Dr. H. C. Cameron of London in a discussion of Byron's lameness before the Royal Society of Medicine on March 21, 1923, is quoted by the *British Medical Journal* as saying: "Moore, his [Byron's] biog-

[1] A part of the amnion, a membrane enveloping the fetus, which occasionally covers the head of a child at birth.

rapher who knew him well; Galt, also his biographer and companion on one of his eastern tours; Lady Blessington and the Countess of Albrizzi, both great friends of his, could never make up their minds which foot was deformed. His boxing instructor, Gentleman Jackson, thought it was his left. His mother, writing to her sister-in-law about taking the opinion of John Hunter, stated definitely, 'It is the right foot.' Mrs. Leigh Hunt, who with her husband was long Byron's guest thought the left foot was shrunken but that it was not club foot."

Dr. Cameron exhibited two surgical boots which he was sure had been made for and worn by Byron. Both boots were for the right foot, but they were adapted to a long, slender foot and not to a clubfoot. The Doctor believed Byron suffered from a mild case of Little's disease, a spastic type of paralysis due usually to incomplete development of the pyramidal tracts of the brain or to brain injury incurred during the birth process.

Dr. James Kemble, writing in the *West London Medical Journal* on "The Lameness of Lord Byron," describes two boots in possession of the publishing firm of John Murray, London, both of which are for the right foot. One was said to have been fitted when the poet was eleven years of age, the other when he was eighteen. The soles of these boots were wedged in a manner indicating that they were intended to compensate a varus type of clubfoot, that is, one in which the sole of the foot turns inward to face the opposite foot. Another boot was believed to have been worn over the corrective boot, which belief, if well founded, may account for some of the confusion with respect to the type of the deformity.

The consensus of medical opinion is that Byron suffered from clubfoot of the equino-varus type involving the right foot. In this condition there is a shortening of the Achilles tendon in addition to the rotation of the foot in its long axis, so that the cripple, in case of moderate deformity, tends to walk on that part of the sole lying immediately behind the third, fourth, and fifth toes. Apart from specific evidence that Byron's deformity was of that type, there is a statistical probability that it was so since approximately 75 per cent of all cases of congenital clubfoot are of the equino-varus variety.

When at the age of ten years Byron succeeded to the peerage through the death of his father, his mother, sensitive about her child's lameness, turned him over to a Nottingham quack named Lavender who placed the foot in a vice-like contraption and tried to twist it forcibly into normal shape. The result of this exceedingly painful treatment was an acute, though probably only temporary, aggravation of the boy's congenital lameness.

It is difficult to estimate the degree of Byron's disability. The corrective boots which have been preserved indicate a moderate degree of deformity and his known athletic ability supports the conclusion that it was not great. He seems, however, to have walked with a perceptible limp. He boxed and played cricket frequently but probably not very well. As might be expected, his swimming ability was little impaired. His reputation for proficiency in that sport was established on May 3, 1810, when he swam the Hellespont in imitation of the love-smitten Leander; but Byron was his own Hero. He wrote: "I plume myself over this achievement more than I could possibly do on any other kind of glory, political, poetical, or rhetorical." During this visit to the Levant he sojourned for some weeks at Patras near Missolonghi, the village which thirteen years later was to be the scene of his destiny, and nearly died of malaria. His recovery was undoubtedly hindered by a self-imposed regimen designed to preserve the slimness of his figure and enhance the delicacy of his features. It consisted of three Turkish baths weekly, the imbibing of large quantities of water tinctured with vinegar, and an exclusive diet of boiled rice.

On January 2, 1815, Byron was married to Anne Isabella Milbanke and after a couple of months the pair settled at Picadilly Terrace, London. About one year after their marriage Lady Byron gave birth to a girl, and no sooner had her ladyship recovered from her confinement than she took her baby with her to the country and, insisting that her husband was insane, refused ever to return to him. It is generally agreed that Lady Byron left her lord because she believed him guilty of incest with his half-sister, Augusta Leigh, daughter of "Mad Jack" Byron by his first wife. Augusta was a guest in the Byron home during the late months of Lady Byron's pregnancy. Quite apart from her ladyship's reason for leaving Byron, there seems to be evidence that an unnatural relationship did exist and that Augusta bore a daughter as a result of it. André Maurois, in his *Byron*, quotes letters from the poet to Lady Melbourne, his confidante, and to Thomas Moore, his trusted friend, containing highly incriminatory passages. He also adduces other circumstantial evidence to make, on the whole, a strong case against the brother and sister.[2]

The British public was scandalized by the revelations and Byron, uncomfortable in the atmosphere of general hostility, fled to Switzerland. There he was joined by Percy Bysshe Shelley and his family, including Claire Clairmont (stepsister of Mary Godwin Shelley), who continued an affair begun with Byron in London the preceding winter. After a few months the Shelleys returned to England taking Claire with them, Byron remaining behind. Eventually came the news that Claire had borne him a daughter. When the child was given into his custody, Byron changed her name from Alba to Allegra and was pleased by the many compliments paid her brightness and beauty. On the few occasions they were together, he found the role of "papa" strange and difficult. The unfortunate little Allegra was placed in an Italian convent by her father, where she died of typhus at the age of five. When Byron received the news of her death, he was beside himself with grief, but his habitual fatalism soon restored his poise.

A description of Byron's personal appearance at the age of twenty-eight is given in the *Dictionary of National Biography* in these words: "Dark brown locks curving over a lofty forehead, grey eyes with long, dark lashes, a mouth and chin of exquisite symmetry are shown in his portraits and were animated by an astonishing mobility of expression varying from apathy to intense passion. His head was small. . . . He had a broad chest, long, muscular arms with white, delicate hands, and beautiful teeth."

Byron had a dual personality of a sort. Instinctively he was tender, sentimental, generous, and just. But his brain told him that life in this world demanded sterner qualities and that the next world held no reward for softer ones. His second self represents

[2] In 1925 John Drinkwater weighed the evidence for and against the charge and declared that guilt was not proved.

an adaptation to reality. He was, therefore, cold, selfish, passionate in an animal sense, and rebellious. In repose he was a commoner, in action an aristocrat. In all situations of physical danger he was a brave man.

In 1823, Byron decided to cast his lot with the Greek patriots who were organizing a rebellion against the Turks. Pursuant to this decision he, with a small party of fellow travelers, which included E. J. Trelawny, Count Pietro Gamba, Dr. Francesco Bruno, and eight servants, set sail for Greece on Friday, July 13, and after numerous delays, reached Missolonghi in the Gulf of Petras on December 30. The longest delay was at Cephalonia where the poet took up his residence on the small island of Metaxata. There he decided to take a side trip to the islet of Ithaca, and while visiting a monastery on the historic isle, he suddenly went berserk and, raving and cursing, chased everybody from the room, barred the doors, and then fell to the floor writhing with abdominal cramps. Dr. Bruno and others carried him to a bed, where, after resting a day and a half, the poet-warrior seemed his normal self. On February 15, 1824, at Missolonghi, while jesting and sipping cider with Parry, his artillery commander, Byron's face suddenly became flushed, his features distorted, and he seemed about to fall. Suddenly, however, the spasm relaxed and he recovered his equilibrium. Subsequently, he declared that he was conscious throughout the episode but had suffered great pain. Dr. Bruno applied leeches to the temples and after withdrawing the leeches had difficulty in stopping the flow of blood.

On April 9, Byron decided to go riding despite the threatening state of the weather. Three miles outside Missolonghi he was drenched by rain. On the return he left his horse and crossed the lagoon to the town in an open boat. By the time he had reached his quarters he was thoroughly chilled. Hot drinks and dry clothing warmed him up, but two hours later he began to shiver and complain of "rheumatic pain." Shortly he remarked to Count Gamba that the pain was more than he could endure. That night he felt feverish and was attended by Dr. Millingen, a German physician in the Greek government service, and Dr. Bruno, his own personal physician. The doctors recommended a hot bath followed by castor oil and antimony internally. The following night he was again very uncomfortable and again slept very little, but the next day he insisted on getting up and going about his duties.

On the afternoon of April 13, his fever was high and the doctors advised him to be bled, but the patient refused and in no uncertain terms denounced the practice of blood-letting. "Have you no other remedy than bleeding?" he asked. "There are more deaths by the lancet than the lance." The doctors expressed the opinion that the symptoms were due to rheumatic fever. During the day of April 14, Byron attended to his affairs, but that night his sleep was disturbed and restless. The following afternoon the fever was high, and again his doctors urged the sick man to submit to bleeding. Again the patient stubbornly refused. Cathartics were administered and he coughed and vomited during the night.

On the morning of the sixteenth, realizing that his condition was steadily worsening, Byron yielded to the advice of the doctors and allowed a pint of blood to be taken. After one hour, no improvement being apparent, he was bled again. For a brief space he seemed better and then was as bad as before. Cold bandages were applied to his head, and Dr. Bruno pleaded for more blood but was refused. The fever increased during the night.

Next morning ten ounces of blood were drawn. The patient sat up and read a little but becoming weak was assisted to his bed. Dr. Treiber, Dr. Millingen's assistant, and Dr. Vaya, physician to Prince Mavrocordato, were called in consultation. Again Bruno clamored for blood, but he was overruled by the other doctors. Shortly after the consultation Byron fainted, his pulse became weak, and his hands and feet grew cold. He was given green tea with laudanum, following which medication he fell asleep. His respiration was jerky and he moaned with each expiration. Leeches were applied to his temples and were thought to have helped. At four o'clock in the afternoon of April 18 he appeared to be sinking and two hours later he fell asleep. He slept all night and the next morning could not be aroused. In the afternoon his respirations grew progressively shallower and faster; at six-fifteen o'clock he died.

A post-mortem examination was made, probably the next morning. Bruno's notes on the findings were amplified by Dr.

Millingen, but even so the report was so sketchy that it threw no light on the cause of death. It was recorded that the cranial sutures were ossified, the dura mater was thick and adherent to the skull, the pia mater was swollen with an exudation of lymph. The brain was congested, the heart was enlarged, flabby, and the ventricular walls thin. The liver was small and hard. No mention was made of the size or appearance of the spleen, which, regardless of the cause of death, must have been altered to some extent if only by malarial attacks years before. The brain condition was probably due to fever and to failing circulation. Apparently the liver changes were those characteristic of cirrhosis.

In 1924 two eminent medical men of Britain, Sir Ronald Ross and Dr. G. C. Low, were handed the clinical records of Byron's final illness and asked to venture a diagnosis. Each, independent of the other, stated that the poet appeared to have died of a virulent type of malarial fever. Sir Ronald implied that the patient's life might have been saved if the physicians had thought to administer cinchona (quinine) and added that whatever the disease may have been, it was surely abetted by the "remorseless bleeding" of the patient and the almost total disregard of the elementary principles of medical care.

In view of the fact that Byron arrived at Missolonghi in midwinter when the malaria-bearing mosquitoes are inactive, it seems likely that he had acquired his infection the previous autumn, probably while resting at Cephalonia, and that it lay dormant through the winter only to leap into activity with the return of warmth and sunshine in the spring. It is extremely unlikely that it had any connection with the malarial attack suffered at Petras thirteen years before.

The maniacal attack at Ithaca and the brief spell of painful immobility experienced on the following February 15 could, conceivably, have been due to explosive flare-ups of smoldering estivo-autumnal malaria. There are, however, rumors of other, similar attacks, suffered prior to those of 1824. The two authenticated attacks, the one at Ithaca and the other at Missolonghi, were almost surely "psychic equivalents" of epileptic seizures. In such attacks the patient may behave as if intoxicated and is likely to become violent, especially if restraint is attempted. Men are affected more often than women, and adults more often than children. Severe abdominal pain such as Byron complained of in the Ithaca episode is rather characteristic.

The common allegation that Byron was epileptic may, therefore, be accepted as essentially true, though, of course, his epilepsy had nothing to do with his death.

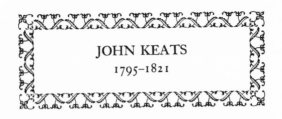

JOHN KEATS
1795–1821

D<small>R. W</small>ILLIAM O<small>SLER</small> in his *An Alabama Student
and Other Essays has given us this eloquent tribute to John Keats:

"All lovers of poetry cherish Keats' memory for the splendor
of the verse with which he has enriched our literature. There is
also that deep pathos of a life cut off in the promise of such rich
fruit. He is numbered among the "inheritors of unfilled renown"
with Catullus, Marlowe, Chatterton, and Shelley whom we mourn
as doubly dead because they died so young."

Keats was the eldest of four children born to a London livery-
stable manager who had been advantageously married to the proprietor's daughter. It is alleged that the poet was born prematurel-
ly, but his biological emancipation, untimely as it may have been,
seems to have imposed no serious handicap, for as a schoolboy he
is said to have been strong, well made, and notably pugnacious.
When he was but fifteen years of age, his mother died of consumption, and shortly thereafter he was apprenticed to Mr. Hammond,
a surgeon at Edmonton. After four years he quarreled with his
mentor and returned to London where he studied at St. Thomas'
and Guy's hospitals. He passed his examination for licentiate in
July, 1816, and seemed on the way to become a successful practitioner when he suddenly decided to devote himself to the art of
the poet.

Through the winter of 1817–18 Keats nursed his brother Tom,
who was waging a losing fight against pulmonary tuberculosis.

The following summer he made a trip to Scotland, and while on the Island of Mull in the West Hebrides, he caught a cold which "settled in his throat." In a letter dated August 6 at Inverness, he describes his throat as "in a fair way of getting well." During the final months of the year he again nursed Tom until the death of the latter in December. On December 31 he complained to Fanny Keats that his sore throat kept him confined to the house and a few weeks later the complaint was repeated.

There is an ominous significance to persistent sore throat in a young person who has been heavily exposed to tuberculosis as Keats was. It is likely to mean laryngeal tuberculosis, a serious and painful disease which occurs rarely except as a complication of tuberculosis elsewhere in the respiratory tract. Until recent years laryngeal tuberculosis was of deadly portent.

In February, 1819, Keats wrote that the sore throat had haunted him for nearly a year. In June and July the trouble was still with him, but after a summer spent on the Isle of Wight and at Winchester, his throat seemed better, though he was dogged by a sense of general ill-being which unfitted him for both physical and mental exertion. He wrote: "I think if I had a free and healthy and lasting organization of heart and lungs as strong as an ox's so as to bear unhurt the shock of an extreme thought and sensation without weariness, I could pass my life nearly alone though it should last eighty years. But I find my body too weak to support me to the height. I am obliged to check myself and be nothing."

During the autumn there was no recorded complaint, but on December 20 he wrote that he feared the winter lest it affect his throat "which on exertion or cold continually threatens me." On February 3, 1820, after a lengthy ride in a stage, he had a spell of bloody expectoration, though apparently there was no free hemorrhage. With the onset of spring the lung symptoms were less evident and, despite his nervous irritability and general weakness, he was able to direct the publication of his third small volume of poems. On June 22 he had a recurrence of bloody expectoration which lasted several days. It was now obvious to the sick man and his physicians that he was beset by a highly dangerous disease. He wrote that it would be a long, tedious affair and that a winter in Italy might be necessary. " 'Tis not yet consumption," he told

Fanny Keats, "but it would be were I to remain in this climate all winter." Accordingly, preparations were made for a journey to Italy which he likens to "marching up to a battery."

After a slow and wearisome voyage, Keats, accompanied by the artist Joseph Severn, landed at Naples near the end of October and then proceeded onward to Rome. Severn has given a pathetic account of the last months of his friend the poet, who, feeling the futility of all efforts to cure his malady, now resolved to end his life. The artist wrote:

> In a little basket of medicine I had bought at Gravesend at his request there was a bottle of laudanum and this, I found, was destined by him to close his mortal career when no hope was left and prevent a long, lingering death for my poor sake. When the dismal time came and Doctor Clark was unable to encounter Keats' penetrating look and eager demand he insisted on having the bottle which I had already put away. Then came the most touching scenes. He now explained to me the exact procedure of his gradual dissolution, enumerated my deprivations and toils and dwelt upon the danger to my life and certainly to my fortunes, from my continued attendance upon him. One whole day was spent in earnest representation of this sort to which, at the same time they wrung my heart to hear and his to utter, I was able to oppose a firm resistance. On the second day his appeal turned to despair in all the power of his ardent imagination and bursting heart.

Dr. Clark and Severn did everything the small medical knowledge of the time and the most devoted affection enabled them to do, but they could neither stay the progress of Keats' malady nor lighten the burden of his despair. Unfortunately, Keats had none of the hopeful attitude of mind characteristically found in the irredeemable victim of consumption—the *spes phthisica* which mirages death in illusory habiliments of joyous life. "I feel," he said, "the flowers growing over me. When will this posthumous life come to an end?"

On February 27 he died peacefully in the arms of the faithful Severn. Only a few days before his death, he had directed that his gravestone should be nameless, bearing only these words:

Here lies one whose name was writ in water.

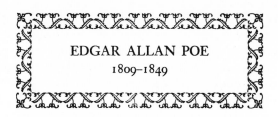

EDGAR ALLAN POE
1809–1849

Lhe tragic life of Edgar Allan Poe, whose brilliance of mind was merged with and eventually absorbed by his madness, would seem to support the theory that genius is sometimes a species of insanity.

Like many another of that group of extraordinary men who distinguished the literary and political life of the American Republic in the first half of the nineteenth century, Poe had Scotch-Irish blood in his veins. His father, Donald Poe, was of pure Scotch-Irish stock; his mother was English.

Donald Poe, who was born in Baltimore, studied law until the lure of the stage abruptly changed the direction of his ambition. As an actor he was strictly of the "ham" variety and while on a visit to New York in 1809, disappeared and was never heard of again. It is quite possible that his disappearance had some connection with his fondness for drink. Edgar's mother, Elizabeth Arnold Poe, who was both beautiful and talented, was cut down at the threshold of a promising stage career when she died at the age of twenty-four. Her death, which occurred in Richmond, Virginia, was caused by pulmonary tuberculosis. She left three children, William Henry Leonard Poe, aged four; Edgar, aged two; and an infant girl named Rosalie. Like his mother, William Henry died of consumption in his twenty-fifth year. Little Rosalie was a backward child who grew up physically but failed to attain

187

mental maturity. She died in an institution for mental defectives at Washington, D. C.

Soon after the death of his mother, Edgar was given a home in the family of John Allan, a Scottish merchant in Richmond, Virginia. Little Eddie was a charming child, handsome, precocious, and friendly. It is said, however, that he was somewhat spoiled by the affectionate attention lavished upon him by Mrs. Allan and a maiden sister who lived in the Allan house. Although the Allans never legally adopted Edgar, their name was incorporated in his, and he was treated, and doubtless regarded, as one of the family until his waywardness won for him the uncompromising enmity of dour old John Allan. Mrs. Allan, however, always had a motherly forgiveness for the peccadilloes of her beloved Eddie.

According to some accounts, when Eddie was four years of age the Allans took him with them to England and Scotland where John Allan spent seven years in answer to the demands of business. The child was sent to several different schools in conformity with the movements of the family. Following their return to Richmond in 1820 Edgar attended the Academy of William Burke and, later, the Joseph H. Clark School. In 1824, at the age of fifteen, he first revealed the morbid side of his nature when he was observed to grieve unnaturally over the insanity and death of Mrs. Stanard, mother of one of his playmates.

At seventeen Edgar matriculated at the University of Virginia and quickly became a figure in the student activities of that famous school. It is noted that he possessed an abundant self-conceit, was socially ambitious, and excelled in language, literature, oratory, and dramatics; but, as is common in persons with strong literary inclinations, he had no taste for mathematics. Because of his classroom brilliance and engaging personality he was a favorite with his teachers. Though considered studious, he found time, it seems, for a little conviviality and a considerable amount of card playing. It is said that he could not "carry his liquor well," and that if he drank at all, he was likely to keep at it as long as the swallowing mechanism continued to function. To the immense disgust of John Allan, Edgar contracted debts which were considerably augmented by futile attempts to repay them with winnings from the gaming table. Allan not only refused to pay the debts of his protégé but also went to Charlottesville and brought the lad back to Richmond and put him to work in the Allan store. The two quarreled continually until Edgar packed his belongings and ran away to Boston where he lived under the name of Henri Le Rennet. There he induced an obscure printer named Thomas to publish his first volume, *Tamerlane and Other Poems*. The edition was small and yielded neither gold nor glory, but it was a beginning.

On May 6, 1827, Poe enlisted in the United States Army under the name of Edgar A. Perry. Records in the Adjutant General's Office show that he claimed to be *twenty-two* years of age, was five feet, eight inches in height, eyes gray, hair brown, and complexion fair. His respiratory movements were free and equal on the two sides, his limbs symmetrical and without deformity. No heart disorder was noted. He was assigned to Battery "H" of the First Artillery. He had a good service record and was discharged with the rank of sergeant major on April 4, 1829. He had to get a substitute before separation from the service could be granted. His superior officers recommended him for West Point.

While awaiting his appointment to the Military Academy, he lived at the home of his aunt, Mrs. Clemm, in Baltimore. Meantime he published another book of poems. In June, 1830, he entered "the Point," where he did very well for a time. Apparently he was able to conquer his distaste for mathematics, for he ranked near the top in the two examinations taken during his cadetship. But after a few months his habitual dissatisfaction with the *status quo* drove him to seek his discharge. The allegation that the superior attitude of his fellow cadets toward a man from the ranks was the spring of his discontent is probably baseless. In a spirit of rebellion he absented himself from minor duties and refused to obey the order of the officer of the day to attend church. He was court-martialed, found guilty, and dismissed from the service of the United States on March 6, 1831. Evidently his infractions were forgiven, for he is now honored by a bronze tablet above the door of the room he occupied during his nine months at the Academy.

The year 1831 was fraught with adversity for the mercurial minded Edgar. He was humiliated by a jail sentence, brief though it was, for a debt of eighty dollars; he developed a running ear and was advised to give up his favorite sport of swimming because of heart trouble. In November he was acutely ill, but the nature of his ailment is not discoverable. About this time, it is said, he began taking opium to tide him over his recurrent fits of depression but broke off the habit before it became fixed, which indicates that his use of the drug could not have been heavy or prolonged. It is possible that pre-addiction to alcohol made the use of opium less attractive for him since it is well established that confirmed alcoholics find little satisfaction in opiates and opium addicts commonly spurn alcohol.

In 1833, Poe addressed a final letter to John Allan in which he begged for sympathy and assistance in the losing war which his conscience was waging against his impulses. He described himself as neither vicious nor licentious, but merely the victim of a deep and inexplicable despondency which seized him periodically and from which drink was his only refuge. And in a letter to J. P. Kennedy a couple of years later Edgar again expressed his incomprehension of his recurring spells of despair which seemed spontaneous and unrelated to external conditions.

At the age of twenty-six Poe was secretly married to his first cousin, Virginia Clemm, aged thirteen. Six months later, after he had gone to Richmond to assume editorship of the *Southern Literary Messenger*, he sent for Virginia and her mother and had a public re-marriage. The bride was a delicate child who failed to develop physically, owing, perhaps, to the presence of chronic pulmonary tuberculosis to which she succumbed ten years later. His attitude toward her was always one of the greatest tenderness. Those who knew the couple best believed that the relationship was actually that of a foster parent to a frail and innocent child.

Under his editorship the *Messenger* flourished surprisingly, but after a few months Edgar went on a protracted spree to appease his melancholy and, as a consequence, was discharged from his job. Upon his promise to drink no more he was rehired some weeks later, but finding himself emerging from a condition of deep insobriety one day, he decided to save face and send in his resignation. From Richmond he returned to New York and the hospitality of his mother-in-law, who had preceded him. It is difficult to see how Poe could have managed to exist during this period without the help of Mrs. Clemm, who was put to every decent extremity to provide a minimum of life's necessities for Virginia, Edgar, and herself. On at least one occasion Edgar left the side of his sick wife to go on a binge in Brooklyn, where he was found days later "wandering about like a crazy man." It appears that it was about this time that the sauce of migrainous headaches was added to his diet of woe.

After a year and a half in New York he took Virginia and Mrs. Clemm with him to Philadelphia, where he went to assume the co-editorship of *Burton's Gentleman's Magazine*. It was a repetition of the old story. For a brief period he did well, but inevitably he got drunk, quarreled with his employer, and quit his job. He had just published two volumes of his work, and the reception accorded them proved that despite the stultifying effects of melancholia and intemperance he was achieving considerable success in the field of literature.

In 1841, Poe enjoyed the brief best months of his confused life. As literary editor of *Graham's Lady's and Gentleman's Magazine* he was influential in making it the most popular periodical of the kind in the United States. In the spring of 1842 he quit *Graham's* in order, apparently, to make drinking and poetry his full-time occupation. After several months of dissipation he dragged his wretched body to the office of a friendly doctor named Mitchell who diagnosed "heart trouble" and paid the costs for a course of treatment at Saratoga Springs. Improved in health, he returned to his wife and her mother in Philadelphia. For the next two years he lectured, loafed, wrote a little, and went on sprees, according to his mood. Late in 1844 he returned to New York.

A remarkable resurgence in 1845 brought him first the editorship and then the proprietorship of the *Broadway Journal*. In the second capacity he progressed brilliantly for about three months, which, owing to the cyclic nature of his mental disorder, was about as long as he could hold an even pace. Then he neglected his work and spent his substance on drink. In the following January his wife died, his health was bad, and he was deeply in debt. He abandoned the *Journal* completely and for months his status was little better than that of a drunken beggar. A year later he had developed paranoid delusions as is revealed in his lectures on Cosmography of the Universe and his plans for the construction of a "thinking machine." He tried to commit suicide by drinking laudanum, but his resistance to the effects of the opiate, enhanced by earlier use of the drug, defeated the venture.

In the latter part of September, 1849, Poe arrived in Baltimore and, it is alleged, promptly fell into the hands of a political gang who plied him with drink and used him as a "repeater" at the polls in a local election held a few days after his coming. At any rate, on the day after the election he was found in a semiconscious condition in a well-known Baltimore tavern by his old friend Dr. James E. Snodgrass, who had instituted a search for him. Dr. Snodgrass had the sick man placed in Washington Hospital under the care of Dr. J. J. Moran. Four days later, in a state of wild delirium, the patient suddenly collapsed and died. The diagnosis was cerebral edema of alcoholic origin.

It is not easy always to separate those incidents in Poe's behavior which were due to inherent insanity from those due to chronic alcoholism. But, taking the larger view, it is easy to see that his mental disease not only preceded but also underlaid his dipsomania. He had his first serious emotional disturbance at the age of fifteen, before he began to drink. Subsequently he declared, plausibly enough, that he resorted to drink only to combat his attacks of despondency. He never tried to place the blame on bad social influences. He was a solitary periodic drinker, a fact of much diagnostic significance.

It is not far wrong to say that all solitary periodic drinkers are basically of Poe's type. It would be wrong, of course, to say that all persons of this basic type are drunkards or even drink at all. Neither are all of them geniuses, though most of them do possess special abilities well above those of the run of men. In general they are the fellows who could achieve brilliant successes if, in the popular phrase, "they would only leave liquor alone."

Psychiatrists agree that Poe suffered from a manic-depressive psychosis with alternating periods of high elation and deep depression. His drunkenness, though it accounted for his death, was merely a symptom of the cyclic mental disease which possessed him for many years. His genius, great as it unquestionably was, came at a high price indeed!

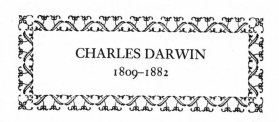

CHARLES DARWIN
1809–1882

THOSE WHO HAVE READ the published letters of Charles Darwin are aware that throughout most of his adult life the great naturalist was plagued by chronic illness. It is generally agreed by medical men that he had a neurotic disposition, but it must be remembered that neuroticism is not a shield against organic disorders, though it may, and very often does, overshadow and obscure the presence of associated physical disease. The story of Darwin's suffering invites our sympathy without by any means satisfying our curiosity with respect to the nature of his ailment.

Apparently he was a strong, healthy young man when at the age of twenty-two he embarked on the famous five-year cruise of H.M.S. *Beagle*. Some months after the return he made his first recorded complaints of ill health. He suffered from a persistent abdominal discomfort so oppressive in character that even the buoyance of a successful courtship could not lift him from the mire of his distress. Sympathetic medical biographers have placed the responsibility for Darwin's broken health on hardships endured in the course of the *Beagle* expedition, a venture which entailed much exposure and discomfort both aboard ship and ashore. Darwin himself tells of his incessant seasickness whenever out of sight of land and his pitiful attempts to arrange and classify collected specimens as the tiny ship was tossed about on the stormy seas of the South Atlantic. A minor cruise of three hundred miles in an open boat off Tierra del Fuego was truly an agonizing experience. With the repeated prolonged attacks of nausea during the five years there undoubtedly went starvation-acidosis and vitamin deprivation of considerable degree. Moreover, while on land he was constantly active, climbing mountains or making long trips on horseback. It is said that he was frequently in the saddle for as long as ten hours without either rest or sustenance.

At the end of the *Beagle* expedition, Darwin took up his residence in London, but because the hurly-burly of the great city seemed to aggravate his ailment, he moved to Down in 1841, resolved to spend the rest of his life in rural quiet and seclusion. There, as time went on, his social, physical, and intellectual activities were increasingly restricted because of the slow but steady deterioration in the state of his health.

Curiously, Darwin's many letters to his intimate friends, especially W. D. Fox and Sir J. D. Hooker, complain of frequent episodes of illness but usually say little or nothing about symptoms. At one time or another, however, they mention attacks of vomiting occasioned by "conversational strain," insomnia, extreme fatigability, headaches, and mental depression, palpitation, and discomfort in the region of the heart, and chronically disordered digestion. In a letter to Sir J. D. Hooker in 1845, Darwin says: "I believe I have not had one day or rather, night, without my stomach having been greatly disordered during the last three years."

He was always extremely sensitive to cold, but evidently he took cold baths not only at Ilkey, where he was accustomed to go for "hydropathy," but also at home, for in a letter to the elder Hooker dated October 12, 1849, he wrote:

> You asked about my cold water cure. I am going on very well and am certainly a little better every month. My nights mend much slower than my days. I have built a douche and am to go on through all the winter, frost or no frost. My treatment now is, lamp four or five times per week and shallow bath for five minutes afterward; douche daily for five minutes and dripping sheet daily. The treatment is wonderfully tonic. . . . the water cure together with three short walks is curiously exhausting and I am forced to go to bed completely tired. I gain steadily in weight and eat immensely and

am never oppressed with my food. I have lost the involuntary twitching of the muscles and all the faint feeling, etc. Doctor Gully thinks he shall quite cure me in six to nine months more.

Unhappily Dr. Gully's hopeful prognosis seems to have failed of realization, for in a letter to W. D. Fox dated March 7, 1852, Darwin wrote, "I dread going anywhere on account of my stomach so easily failing under my excitement." And in October of the same year he wrote from his home in Down, "The other day I went to London and back and the fatigue, though so trifling, brought on my bad form of vomiting." Five years later found him at Moor Park, Farnham, "undergoing hydropathy for a fortnight." He wrote, "I can not in the least understand how hydropathy can act as it certainly does on me. It dulls one's brain splendidly."

His daily routine, thought to have been prescribed by Sir Andrew Clark, was as follows: 7:45, breakfast; 8–9:30, work in the study; 12:30, luncheon; 1:30–2:00, rest in the recumbent posture; 2–3:00, writing letters; 3–4:00, napping in bed; 4–4:30, walk in the open air; 4:30–5:30, work in the study; 6–7:00, rest in bed reading aloud; 7:00, light supper; 8–10:00, games, reading, etc., in drawing room; 10:30, to bed. This schedule, it will be noted, allows for five hours of work, including letter writing; the remainder of the day was to be spent in some manner designed to safeguard his health. Eight and one-half hours were spent in bed at night. There were, however, many periods when for weeks at a time he felt unable to do any work at all. Nevertheless, he managed, in a life of semi-invalidism, to write not less than twenty-two separate works of importance. Perhaps it was because of a disquieting anxiety to get his ideas into print that his literary style is generally involved and difficult of understanding. He himself said he never could learn to write fluent, lucid English, but the admirable clarity of occasional passages in his works indicates that with care he could have written better than he did.

For thirty-four years his life was a wearisome monotony of ill health, suffering, and despondency. Then, about 1872, there began an abatement of his symptoms which brought "great satisfaction and hope" to his family. From this time on his physical and nervous discomforts underwent a gradual amelioration, though there was an intensification of his sense of weakness. In 1881 he commenced to have attacks of angina pectoris due, probably, to sclerotic disease of the coronary arteries. Early the following year evidences of cardiac decompensation first appeared, and on April 19, 1882, he expired.

Much has been written on the neurosis of Charles Darwin. In 1845 in a letter to J. D. Hooker, Darwin made this significant statement: "Many of my friends, I believe, think me a hypochondriac." It was true, indeed, that many of his friends did think him a hypochondriac, and their belief has been shared since then by many medical men who have expressed their conviction and the reasons therefor in the literature of the profession. Apparently the neuropsychiatrists have claimed the great evolutionist for their own and the gastroenterologists are disposed to concede them the right of proprietorship. For example, Dr. Edward J. Kempf in the *Psychoanalytic Review* advances the concept that Darwin suffered from a "father complex" and could have benefited by modern psycho-therapy.

That Darwin had a neurotic constitution is abundantly evident. First of all there was his ready susceptibility to seasickness, a tendency which denotes a high-strung, sensitive nervous system. That mere fatigue or conversational strain should set off an attack of vomiting even in the presence of a demonstrable gastric lesion would show a psychoneurotic background. And that a series of cold baths which "dull one's brain splendidly" should relieve the "involuntary twitching of muscles" and enable him to "eat immensely" and never be "oppressed with my food" would seem not only to prove his neurosis but, at the same time, to rule out any sort of concomitant organic gastric disorder.

In his book, *Nervousness, Indigestion, and Pain*, Dr. Walter C. Alvarez, eminent gastroenterologist of the Mayo Clinic, devotes some space to a consideration of the heredity of Darwin as the key to an explanation of the asthenia of the great naturalist. Says Dr. Alvarez: "Back in 1912 when I began to try to understand the problems of the asthenic I learned much about their disease through reading *The Life and Letters of Charles Darwin*. There I found the story of a man who for forty years suffered terribly from weakness, fatigue, headache, insomnia, sinking feelings, and dizzi-

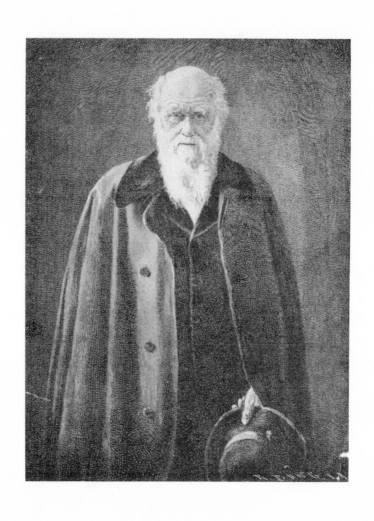

CHARLES DARWIN

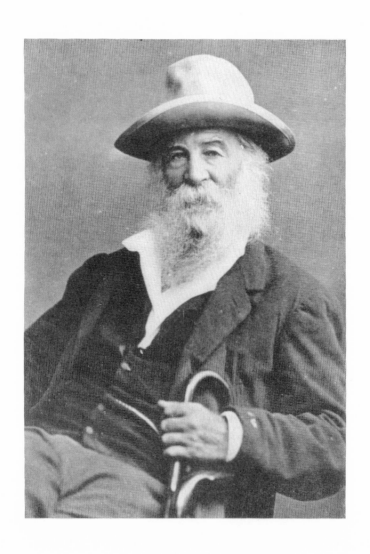

WALT WHITMAN

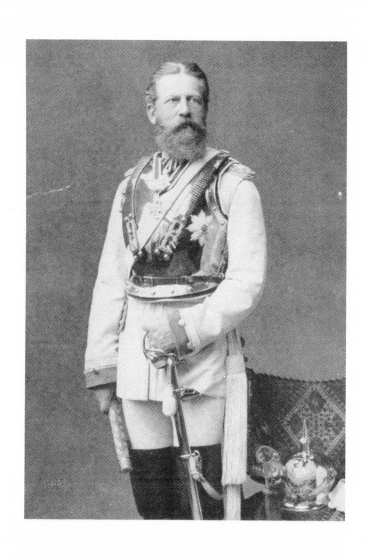

FREDERICK III OF PRUSSIA

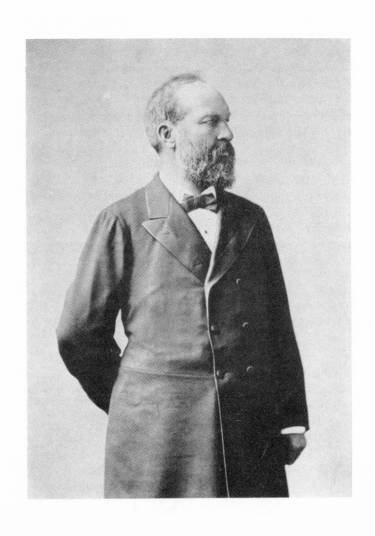

JAMES A. GARFIELD

ness. It was an effort to walk or even to hold up a book. Work and excitement always made him worse, while resting brought some relief."

After citing numerous excerpts from *The Life and Letters of Charles Darwin,* Alvarez continues: "The fact that no physician could ever find anything physically wrong with Darwin and the fact that up until the last few days of his 73 years he never developed symptoms of any organic disease make it fairly certain that his troubles were functional and due to an inherited peculiarity of the nervous system. As soon as I learned that extreme degrees of asthenia such as Darwin suffered from are common equivalents of melancholia, I started hunting through the biographies of the Darwin and Wedgwood families [Darwin's mother was Susannah Wedgwood] to see if I could find such heredity, and there it was. Much of the nervous defect probably came through Charles' paternal grandfather, the famous Dr. Erasmus Darwin who stammered badly and in other ways was odd. A strain of weakness may have come also from Erasmus' first wife who was always sickly, and died at the age of 30. Their first son, Charles, stammered. The second son, Erasmus, was a listless, hypersensitive, and melancholy dreamer who finally committed suicide. His father is reported to have called him 'that poor insane coward.' The third son, Robert, the father of the great Charles Darwin, was able but 'sensitive to an abnormal degree.'

"As if this nervous heredity were not bad enough, Charles Darwin inherited a tendency to melancholia also from his mother's stock. According to Pearson, her father had at least one short nervous breakdown. One of her brothers, Tom Wedgwood, suffered terribly from fits of depression with great abdominal distress. According to Litchfield, his biographer, toward the close of his short life his condition was hardly distinguishable from insanity.

"Tom's two sisters failed to marry. The younger one, Sarah, was described as having a difficult nature, very sensitive, very rigid, and with strong views as to how others should conduct themselves.

"As one would expect with this poor nervous heredity on both sides, the famous Charles Darwin was not the only child to suffer. His brother Erasmus was, according to West, 'An odd figure, a quiet passive personality.' No stronger than Charles constitutionally, he lived 'in patient idleness,' and never worked. In his later years he developed a 'fundamental melancholy.' A sister, Catharine, 'had neither good health nor good spirits' and did not marry until she was 53.'

"With so much nervous ill health in the family it is remarkable that Charles Darwin's children were as well as they were. Apparently Sir George Darwin had ill health all his life and one child failed to develop mentally."

Mention has already been made of Sir Andrew Clark, who was Charles Darwin's personal physician in the later years of the latter's life. In this connection Sir Charles Darwin wrote: "It was not only for his generously rendered service that my father felt a debt of gratitude towards Sir Andrew Clark. He owed to his cheering personal influence an oft-repeated encouragement, which latterly added something real to his happiness, and he found sincere pleasure in Sir Andrew's friendship and kindness towards himself and his children."

Dr. Alvarez concludes: "It should be a comfort to the many ambitious asthenics to know that in spite of the terrible handicap which prevented Darwin from working more than a few hours a day, he was able to accomplish much; his 22 published volumes fill a fair sized shelf, his knowledge of scientific literature was encyclopedic, and as everyone knows, he changed the thought of the world."

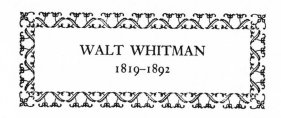

WALT WHITMAN
1819–1892

With the publication of his sensational *Leaves of Grass* in 1855, Walt Whitman may be said to have added a new dimension to the form of poetry. Certainly he presented a metrical and stylistic concept unknown theretofore to the art of poetics. Both the substance and the mechanics of *Leaves of Grass* met with much stormy weather, but it is now generally conceded that Whitman's high place among the immortals of literature is secure.

Walt was accustomed to describe himself as the living definition of robustiousness, "One of the roughs, large, proud, affectionate, eating, drinking, and breeding, his costume manly and free, his face sunburnt and bearded, his posture strong and erect. . . . If health were not his distinguishing attribute, this poet would be the very harlot of persons."[1] Perhaps the depiction can be made to do for the years of his young manhood, but beyond there it does not fit at all.

Whitman was born at West Hills, Long Island, May 31, 1819, the second of nine children. His father, Walter Whitman, was a powerfully built, quiet, industrious man, a Hicksite Quaker, small farmer, and carpenter. His mother, Louisa Van Velsor Whitman, was of mixed Dutch and Welsh blood, comely in her younger days, and always devoted to her family. Neither parent had any interests beyond the pressing problems of making a living and

[1] From one of Walt's own anonymous reviews of his *Leaves of Grass*.

199

rearing their children. Walter Whitman died at the age of sixty-six of paralysis due to cerebral hemorrhage; Louisa died at seventy-eight of causes unknown. The first child, a boy, is said to have been mentally deficient. He died of syphilis of the circulatory and nervous systems at the age of fifty-two. The youngest child was feeble minded and epileptic; he died at the age of fifty-six or fifty-seven of valvular heart disease. Of the others, it appears that at least two died of pulmonary tuberculosis.

When Walt was four years of age, the family moved to Brooklyn, where in due time he was sent to the public schools. At the age of thirteen his formal education ended and he went to work, first as a printer's devil, then a doctor's errand boy, and next as a typesetter apprentice. At eighteen he became a school teacher, but after two years he returned to the print shop, this time as editor of his own paper, *The Long Islander*, in the town of Huntington. Shortly, however, he gave up the paper and returned to Brooklyn, where, after frivoling briefly with another paper, he was given the editorship of the *Brooklyn Eagle*. On the side he wrote articles, stories, and poems for other publications. In 1842 he wrote a temperance novel under the trionym of *Franklin Evans: or The Inebriate: A Tale of the Times*, stipulating anonymity for the author that he might feel free to take a drink when he wanted it.

In 1848, having lost his position as editor of the *Eagle*, he journeyed to New Orleans to assume editorship of the *Crescent*, a post which he filled without great distinction either to himself or to his paper. But he greatly enjoyed the mellow gaiety and the easy living of the hospitable city. It is said that his sojourn at New Orleans amounted to exactly three months, though in after years he was wont to give the impression that he had stayed much longer. He claimed that he had found the queen of sweetness and beauty in the old town, that he had sired six children there, and that altogether he had had a most marvelous experience. Manifestly on the occasions of such talk he was merely indulging his penchant for romantic fancies.

In his maturity Walt was tall and heavy, but he was not the powerful and rugged fellow he claimed himself. John Burroughs said of Whitman that his body "was that of a child" and there was always "something fine, womanly, and delicate in him." He was fond of cooking and bathing and as a young man inclined to be dandyish. After his return from New Orleans he affected the rough dress which he believed comported best with the type of character he aspired to be. For many years he wore regularly an enormous stud of pearls upon the bosom of his open-throated shirt. He drank moderately but never smoked, bathed his face several times daily in eau de cologne, and preferred the company of men to that of women. He was never married. In 1849 he had his cranial topography surveyed at the Fowler and Wells phrenological cabinet, where he was pronounced a many-sided genius of the first rank. This "scientific" confirmation of Walt's somewhat tentative estimate of his own abilities gave his ego a tremendous bounce. He now felt free to obey every internal impulse secure in the knowledge that it flowed from the fountainhead of infallibility.

When the first volume of *Leaves of Grass* was published, Walt wrote anonymously several extravagantly laudatory reviews of the work and its author. These were published in the *Brooklyn Times*, the *American Phrenological Journal*, and the *United States Democratic Review*. It is said that he wrote at least half of John Burroughs' praiseful *Notes on Walt Whitman as Poet and Person.* Walt's apparent self-esteem probably had in it more of animal exuberance than conceit. Whatever it was, it held not the slightest trace of either arrogance or aloofness. All who knew him agree that he was the friendliest and most likable of men.

The first literary authority to pass favorable judgment on *Leaves of Grass* was Ralph Waldo Emerson, who addressed a letter to Whitman declaring, "I find it the most extraordinary piece of wit and wisdom that America has yet contributed. . . . I greet you at the beginning of a great career." The Sage of Concord regretted his rashness when a second edition, widely denounced as pornographic, appeared bearing his encomium on the backstrip.

Walt lived in Brooklyn at the home of his brother, Andrew Jackson Whitman, in the years immediately preceding the outbreak of the Civil War. It was during this period that he suffered what was believed to be a sunstroke, but which was probably a small cerebral hemorrhage. He recovered rather quickly and his health was good except for the occasional bad colds which harried him all his life. He divided his time between his profession of writing and his hobby of visiting sick and disabled omnibus drivers in the Old New York Hospital. Then one day in December, 1862, word came that his brother George, a Union soldier, had been wounded in Burnside's bloody defeat by Lee on the Rappahannock near Fredericksburg. Walt left for the front immediately. Upon his arrival he found that George's injury was not serious but that there was a great need for help in caring for men who had been badly wounded. Walt remained at Fredericksburg for several weeks, doing what he could for the suffering and dying men crowded into the big brick house which had been converted into an emergency hospital. In January, Walt went to Washington determined to remain there indefinitely to work with the war casualties filling the hospitals, regular and makeshift, in the nation's capital. In June he had a severe attack of sore throat with high fever and great pain in the throat and head; a month later, while helping a surgeon to amputate a gangrenous leg, Walt accidentally punctured a hand on the point of the operator's knife. Infection ensued, the hand became painful, and red streaks ran up the arm, denoting inflammation of the lymphatic vessels of the skin. He wished to continue at his work as hospital orderly, but the doctors would not hear to it. After the acute symptoms of his infection had subsided, he was sent home with instructions to remain there for six months. During his vacation he suffered from a fullness in his head with frequent headaches, all of which he ascribed to exposure to the sun.

After Walt had returned to Washington and his hospital work in January, 1864, he was well except for occasional sensations of "fullness in the head" and attacks of faintness. These annoying symptoms increased both in frequency and severity until mid-July when he was "prostrated," undoubtedly by a small cerebral hemorrhage. It would have been informative to have had a blood pressure reading at this time, but the sphygmomanometer was not in common clinical use until thirty years later. It is likely that his blood pressure was somewhat elevated but unlikely that it was very high. Certainly the capillaries and the smallest arteries of the brain were in a condition of fragility, the result of degenerative changes, and it was this condition that prompted the headache and fullness of the head which caused him so much discomfort. He continued to have occasional small strokes until the autumn of 1869 when he was stricken so severely that he was partially paralyzed. He recovered well, however, and remained in reasonably good condition until January 4, 1873, when he awoke one night to find his left arm and leg partially paralyzed. The leg was worse involved than the arm—the face and organs of speech hardly at all.

Under the care of Dr. W. B. Drinkard of Washington, who gave him general care and electrical stimulation of the paralyzed limbs, Walt soon felt well enough to return to the Jersey shore, but he became worse on the way and was taken to the home of his brother George in Camden. He was now cared for by Dr. Matthew J. Grier of Philadelphia and showed gradual improvement until July, 1885, when he had another stroke of such severity that a year later he was "scarcely able to get up and down stairs." About this time a Canadian physician, Dr. Ralph M. Bucke, who was a great friend of Walt's, took the illustrious Dr. William Osler to see the sick poet. Dr. Osler gave Walt a careful examination and told him that "the machine was in fairly good condition considering the length of time it had been on the road." The year 1888 brought another severe stroke, and again Dr. Bucke took Dr. Osler to see the stricken poet. They found him bedfast, mentally confused, and his speech "blurred and indistinct." But improvement occurred to so remarkable a degree that after the lapse of one year he exhibited no trace of either paralysis or speech disturbance.

On March 18, 1891, Dr. Daniel Longaker of Philadelphia examined Walt at the request of the ever faithful Doctor Bucke. The patient was the personification of senility. He looked older than his seventy years, he was barely able to get about with the assistance of a cane, his memory for recent events was poor, and he complained of indigestion, constipation, and "bladder trouble." His heart and lungs seemed in good condition, however, and there was not much hardening of palpable arteries. Massage, laxatives, and catheterization were prescribed and there was some amelioration of symptoms, probably without organic improvement.

On the afternoon of December 17, 1891, Whitman had a severe chill with a rise of temperature to 102 degrees. There was some hoarseness and he coughed up mucous tinged with pus. Prostration was severe and loss of appetite complete. Obviously an acute infection had supervened. Physical examination indicated areas of consolidation in both lungs, but more in the right than in the left. It was believed that he had "a widely diffused bronchopneumonia." The heart seemed to be slowly weakening, and by the fourth day there was a rattle in the windpipe and the lips and finger tips were bluish. At the end of the first week it was noted that the lung involvement had spread, the respiration was labored, and the pulse was rapid and weak. Two days later the patient was stuporous but could be roused easily. Although the pulse was still weak and irregular, there was an impression of faint improvement in the general condition. By December 29 it was evident that the day of exodus was not yet at hand, and accordingly a professional nurse, Mrs. Elizabeth Keller, was called on the case. By January 7, pulse and respirations were normal and all alarming symptoms had subsided.

Two months later he was still bedfast, and it was observed that if he turned on his right side, there was an immediate outburst of coughing with profuse expectoration. The doctors reasoned he must have a large cavity in one lung so situated that accumulated mucous drained out when a posture favorable for its evacuation was assumed. The general condition of the patient showed a downward trend. He was greatly troubled by hiccough and it was impossible for him to find a comfortable position even for a few minutes. Both bladder and bowel function were badly impaired. On March 23 it was noted that his breathing was becoming increasingly difficult and the pulse was weak and faltering. On March 26, 1892, without sound or struggle, the vapor of life deserted the body of Walt Whitman.

Over the violent protests of Mrs. Davis, the Whitman housekeeper, a post-mortem examination was made. Dr. Henry W. Cattell, demonstrator of gross morbid anatomy in the University of Pennsylvania Medical School, conducted the examination. The principal findings were, for the most part, unexpected. It was recorded that "Both the head and brain were remarkably well formed and symmetrical . . . and the brain substance was excessively soft." The weight of the brain was 45 ounces, 292.5 grains avoirdupois, which is almost exactly 4 ounces less than the average for the brain of a normal adult male. The disparity was, no doubt, due to atrophy which, in turn, was the result of cerebral arteriosclerosis of long standing and severe grade. The heart was flabby but otherwise not remarkable. Death, it was revealed, was occasioned by advanced tuberculosis of the right lung, collapse of the left lung, tuberculous empyema, left, fistulous connection of left pleural cavity with a bronchial tube, and disseminated abdominal tuberculosis. Other findings considered noncontributory to death were tuberculous abscesses of sternum, fifth rib, and left foot; a single large gallstone, cyst of an adrenal gland, prostatic hypertrophy, cerebral arteriosclerosis, cloudy swelling of kidneys.

The source of Whitman's tuberculosis was probably within his own family, and it is likely that the germs were implanted in one or both lungs during his childhood or early adolescence. The fact that his mother complained of "soreness and distress in my side" and "bad coughing" suggests that she may have harbored the disease in her chest. It will be recalled that at least two of the Whitman brothers besides Walt are thought to have had pulmonary tuberculosis.

Because of his predilection for the company of men, his habit of addressing young men in terms of endearment, his curious bodily attributes, and finally, perhaps, what John Burroughs termed "the nudity of his verse," Whitman has often been suspected of sexual perversion. The suspicion, however, has never been substantiated. Dr. Josiah C. Trent, of Durham, North Carolina, whose case history of Walt Whitman is the source of the medical data used in this article, says, "By no standards could Whitman's attitude and behavior toward sex be considered 'normal.'" Dr. Trent then quotes John Burroughs on the infantile configuration of Whitman's body and the delicate texture of his skin, and inclines to relate the poet's physical peculiarities to his personality. In conclusion the Doctor employs the interrogatory method to make a provocative suggestion: "Could he," asks Dr. Trent, "have been eunuchoid?"

Unfortunately for the quality of human curiosity, the body we would re-examine for the final answer is dust and the soul we would search has departed this world. But—

Praised be the fathomless universe
For life and joy, and for objects and knowledge curious
And for love, sweet love—but praise! praise! praise!
For the sure en-winding arms of cool-enfolding death.

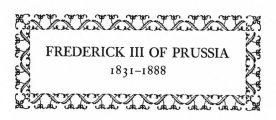

FREDERICK III OF PRUSSIA
1831–1888

F REDERICK III, father of the late Kaiser Wilhelm II of Germany, was born near Potsdam and educated at the University of Bonn. His early life was uneventful.

In 1858, while still crown prince, he was married to the eldest daughter of Queen Victoria of England. He was already known as a strong Liberal, and this event "increased his admiration for English Parliamentary Government even as it secured the silent blessing of England for German unity."

In a quick succession of wars with Denmark, Austria, and France, Frederick displayed great personal courage as well as military ability of the first order. He opposed the high-handed methods of Bismarck, but in his junior position was powerless against the Iron Chancellor. He was tremendously popular with the subject people who looked forward to his accession with the most hopeful expectations.

His health was always good until 1886, when he suffered an attack of measles which left him with a persistent hoarseness, an annoying cough, and an unwonted depression of spirits. On March 6, 1887, the laryngologist, Professor Gerhardt, examined Frederick's throat and discovered an excrescence on the left vocal cord. Gerhardt "attempted to remove the growth by a wire snare and a circular knife, but without success because of the hardness, smoothness and flatness of the lesion. He then tried cauterization. After thirteen applications of an incandescent wire, the growth had entirely disappeared and at its site there was an uneven, reddish, granulated surface at the edge, April 7, 1887."

Re-examination on May 15 disclosed that the growth had recurred and was larger than before cauterization. Professor Ernst von Bergmann of Berlin was called in consultation. Three days later it was agreed by all in attendance that the Crown Prince had cancer and that the larynx should be split (laryngotomy) to permit removal of the growth-bearing vocal cord and adjacent tissues.

Chances of his surviving the operation were fairly good, but only if it were done very early would there be a chance of a lasting cure. There was official hesitation to subject the royal patient to so considerable a risk of life, to say nothing of certain loss of voice.[1] It was decided, therefore, to seek the opinion of some world-famous laryngologist. There were political as well as medical considerations.

After prolonged discussion the choice fell upon Morell Mackenzie, eminent British throat specialist, who examined Frederick's larynx, but refused to concur in the diagnosis of cancer in the absence of microscopic evidence of malignancy. Three particles of the growth were removed by Mackenzie and turned over to Rudolph Virchow, "father" of the new science of cellular pathology. Virchow could find no indication of cancer, the British specialist was given management of the case, and the discredited but unconvinced German doctors awaited the verdict of time.

At the insistence of Queen Victoria, who argued that the summer climate of London is more salubrious than that of Berlin, Frederick departed for the English capital, where, at the Royal Palace, he was daily under the watchful eye of his doctor. When he announced that he had performed an operation on Frederick's throat, using cocaine as a local anesthetic, and had removed what appeared to be all of the growth, Mackenzie seemed to have justified the royal trust. He was joyfully acclaimed at home and abroad and on September 7 was knighted by Queen Victoria. He was at high noon in his day of glory.

---

[1] Persons deprived of the vocal cords or larynx commonly learn to speak in a peculiar whisper produced by combined action of cheeks, tongue, and lips. A "sound box" has recently been devised which has made enunciation possible for these unfortunates.

Frederick journeyed to San Remo, Italy, to escape the rigors of the oncoming German winter. Mackenzie followed shortly and on November 6 made another inspection of the growth. "Its appearance," he wrote, "was altogether unlike the one I had destroyed and the other swellings which from time to time had shown themselves in the larynx; it had, in fact, a distinctly malignant look . . . without rising from my chair I informed his Majesty that a very unfavorable change had taken place in his throat. He said, 'Is it cancer?' to which I replied, 'I am sorry to say, Sir, it looks very much like it but it is impossible to be certain.' "

Mackenzie then called a consultation of all the physicians who had been connected with the case. They decided that the larynx should be removed, but the disheartened Crown Prince demurred. On February 8, 1888, breathing became so difficult that death by suffocation impended. But Bramann, von Bergmann's assistant, who was standing by for just such an emergency, performed a tracheotomy and inserted a tube into the windpipe below the level of the obstruction. Immediate relief was obtained.

On March 9, 1888, Emperor William I died at the age of 91, and the Crown Prince returned to Berlin, where on March 11 he was proclaimed Emperor Frederick III. It was apparent to all that his reign would be a short one.

On the night of April 13, the Emperor developed a temperature of 103 degrees F. and much pus was discharged from the tracheotomy tube. On June 13 there were signs of a "terminal" pneumonia. On June 15, ninety-nine days after he had ascended the throne, death came to the harassed Emperor. His passing was widely deplored. In the language of Dr. Ficarra, from whose account much of this material was taken, "He aroused the world's best expectations by his goodness and wisdom. In battle he displayed marked bravery; in illness he suffered as heroically as he had fought."

The next day, at Bismarck's request, Mackenzie turned in a complete report of the case. The Chancellor ordered an immediate autopsy which was performed by Virchow. The report on the post-mortem findings has been criticized as incomplete, probably because the abridgment released for publication contained only positive findings. It stated that the Emperor's larynx was extensively involved in a malignant process which had the characteristic features of carcinoma. Secondary growths (metastases) were found in the lymph nodes of the neck. Numerous small abscesses were present in the lower lobes of the lungs.

While the body was yet lying in state, a storm of denunciation was loosed by the German doctors whose early diagnosis of the case had been superseded by the fatal optimism of Sir Morell Mackenzie. The Germans, jealous, resentful, and, most important, *right* in their contention that the growth was malignant, attacked Sir Morell unmercifully. The latter insisted that the growth had turned cancerous after his first examination and hinted that the treatment applied by the German doctors was to blame. Mackenzie argued his case imprudently in a book entitled *The Fatal Illness of Frederick the Noble*, which won for the author official censure by the Royal College of Surgeons (England).

There can be no reasonable doubt that the growth was malignant from the start and that Mackenzie erred in relying upon the new science of microscopic pathology to the exclusion of clinical experience. Virchow, with scientific caution, had reported examination of the tissue to be negative for malignancy, but emphasized that he could not be held responsible for the selection and removal of the specimens brought to him for examination. He would not be a whipping boy for Mackenzie. In June, 1887, he had written that "the healthy condition of the tissue on section warranted a very favorable prognosis, but it was impossible to say whether the particles of tissue *represented the entire morbid process (Erkrankung)*. However, there was nothing present in them which would be likely to arouse suspicion of further, graver disease."

In a mood of speculation it is easy to charge Mackenzie's error with the most tragic consequences, for if the operation of laryngotomy had been done when first advised by the German surgeons, it is quite possible that Frederick would have lived out the years of his heritage. Had he lived as long as did his father, William I, or his son, William II, he would have been on the German throne through the fateful first fourteen years of the twentieth century and the recent course of world history might well have been a happier one.

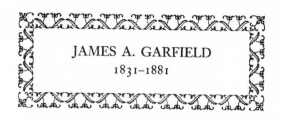

JAMES A. GARFIELD
1831–1881

A T NINE-THIRTY O'CLOCK on the morning of July
2, 1881, in the Baltimore and Potomac railway station at Washington, D. C., James Abram Garfield, twentieth president of the United States, was shot twice by a disappointed officeseeker named Charles Guiteau. At the first shot the President turned to the right and at the second fell to his knees. His assailant was seized before he could fire again, as he might have done since the weapon was a five-chambered, fully loaded revolver. It was of forty-four caliber English bulldog pattern, a deadly instrument at close range.

Mr. Garfield lay face up full length on the floor until a mattress could be procured. Then, with the mattress for a stretcher, he was carried to a room in the second story of the station. A number of doctors, including Surgeon General Barnes and Surgeon Woodward of the army, Dr. D. W. Bliss of Washington, and Dr. Robert Reyburn of New York, were summoned. Immediately after the shooting, the President's pulse was slow and weak, there was a mounting pallor of his cheeks, and his respiration was slow and sighing. Plainly, he was in a state of shock. He complained only of a sense of heaviness in the lower extremities and tingling in the feet. Brandy and aromatic spirits of ammonia were administered by mouth but were rejected by the stomach as the wounded man vomited copiously. Examination revealed that the first bullet had merely grazed the right upper arm, but the second had entered the back four inches to the right of the spinal column on a level with the space between the eleventh and twelfth ribs. It was thought it had ranged forward and downward. At ten-thirty A.M., Mr. Garfield was removed to the White House.

During the next ten hours symptoms of internal hemorrhage were added to those of shock, and several times the patient appeared to be dying. He vomited frequently, and following the spasms of vomiting, he sometimes seemed lifeless for several minutes. Responding in his better moments to the surgeons' inquiries, he stated that the only real pain felt was in his legs and feet. He asked anxiously about his wife, who was hurrying from Elbernon, New Jersey, and he expressed the fear that he might lose consciousness before her arrival. When Mrs. Garfield came in at six–forty-five P.M., the President immediately asked all others to leave the room. After about five minutes she opened the door and requested the doctors and nurses to return to her husband's side. About eight-thirty P.M., it was observed that the patient seemed a little stronger and the doctors were hopeful that the internal bleeding had stopped of its own accord.

Throughout the night the President's stomach tolerated water better and the quality of his pulse improved. By noon of the second day it was apparent that the hemorrhage had ceased. Evidently, as the blood pressure dropped because of diminished blood volume, the flow lessened and clotting occurred at the bleeding points. Under the circumstances it was probably fortunate that the patient could not retain fluids which might have diluted the blood and delayed the process of coagulation.

President Garfield's career had been an inspiring one. He was born in a log cabin near Orange, Ohio, on November 19, 1831. His father died in 1833, leaving a widow and four small children, of which James was the youngest. His boyhood was spent under the harsh conditions of frontier life. He worked hard on the farm to help support the family, attended school three months each winter, and read avidly every book he could buy or borrow. At the age of sixteen he left home to become a canal-boat driver and later the steersman of a boat on the Ohio canal. After several months in this employment he was stricken with malarial fever and forced to relinquish his job and return to his home. Following his recovery he enrolled at Hiram Institute, now Hiram College, in his native state. In due time he entered Williams College, Massachusetts, from which he was graduated with high honors. Returning to Hiram, he taught ancient languages and the classics for a time, after which he became president of the Institute. In his spare moments he studied law and was admitted to the Ohio bar in 1859. Resigning the presidency of Hiram Institute, he was elected to the Ohio State Senate, from which he took his leave to join the army of the North at the beginning of the Civil War.

He was commissioned lieutenant colonel and placed in charge of a regiment made up largely of former students of Hiram Institute. With little time for training, the regiment fought and won an isolated engagement against a vastly greater force of Confederate troops in eastern Kentucky. For this first encounter with the enemy, Colonel Garfield received official commendation for his display of tactical skill and personal bravery. He continued the career so auspiciously begun, and before the end of the war advanced to the rank of major general. Soon after his discharge from the army, he was elected to Congress, where he remained until 1880 when he was chosen president of the United States.

It can be justly said of him that he rose entirely by his own exertions and filled each of his various offices with loyalty, ability, and dignity. He was a large, robust man, over six feet in height and weighing more than two hundred pounds. His habits were temperate and his manner was candid but friendly.

The public reaction to the crime was one of widespread sympathy and indignation. By July 4, two days after the shooting, news of the critical wounding of the President had penetrated to almost every village and farm in the United States. The people of the nation, who assembled in the traditional manner for observance of Independence Day, thought and talked of nothing but the attempt on the life of the President. Hourly bulletins were issued by the attending physicians, and as the reports came off the wires in the local telegraph offices they were sped to the parks and groves where crowds of subdued and anxious citizens were waiting to hear them. The customary programs of amusement and sport were generally suspended as prayers were offered for the President's recovery.

Many persons spent the entire day at the railroad stations,

213

where, in the small communities, the telegraph offices were invariably located. Some of the Civil War veterans branded the attack "another rebel plot." Other citizens, taking note of the assailant's name and being less specific in their antagonisms, assumed that it was the act of "some crazy foreigner." At the end of the day all returned to their homes much heartened by reports of steady improvement in the President's condition. The White House was deluged with telegrams and in the late evening it was announced that Mr. Garfield was greatly cheered by the people's expressions of sympathy and affection.

On July 3 pain in the legs and feet was still so severe as to require morphine injections for relief. The next day pain was nearly gone, though the feet remained sensitive to the touch. There was little nausea or vomiting. The temperature was slightly elevated and the function of the bowels and bladder was uncontrolled. On July 8 a small amount of pus appeared at the opening of the wound in the back and the President's temperature rose to 102.8 degrees. There was nearly continuous moderate fever, and on July 21 a small operation was performed to facilitate drainage. Three days later, following a severe chill the previous evening, the opening of the wound was further enlarged. One of the surgeons pressed his hand against the patient's abdomen and a peculiar white pus welled out of the wound. Following this operation, the fever abated and the President seemed better.

About this time Dr. Alexander Graham Bell, inventor of the telephone, came forward with an instrument designed to ascertain the location of the bullet "in the President's person." The device consisted of a battery, two coils of insulated wire, a circuit breaker, and a telephone. The ends of the primary coil were connected with the battery and those of the secondary coil with the telephone. The coils were so placed in relation to each other that a state of balance was obtained and, consequently, no sound was made by the circuit breaker. A bullet like that within the President's body would, if brought within a few inches of the most sensitive point on the pair of coils, cause a "faint protest against the disturbance" to become audible in the telephone. With these facts established, attempts were made to determine the position of the bullet.

At the appointed time Dr. Bell and an assistant appeared at the White House. Mr. Garfield, bolstered up in bed, watched the proceedings with mute interest. Dr. Bell, holding the telephone to his ear, stood with his back to the patient while his assistant moved the coils over that part of the abdomen where the missile was thought to lie. When the sensitive center of the instrument was immediately over the black-and-blue spot which appeared on the President's abdomen shortly after he was wounded, Dr. Bell cried, "Stop! There it is." The experiment was repeated several times, once with Mrs. Garfield at the telephone, and she heard the "tell-tale singing sound." It was decided that the bullet was somewhat to the right of and about four and one-half inches below the umbilicus. The feeling was that if the time should come when removal of the bullet was desirable, the operation could be undertaken with much greater confidence—thanks to the induction-balance invention of Dr. Bell.

On August 6, to the dismay of all, the fever returned. Another, more extensive operation was deemed advisable. On August 9, under ether anesthesia, a pocket of pus was opened widely. The results seemed to promise well, but nausea and vomiting persisted. Rectal feedings of egg-yolk bouillon, milk, whisky, and a little opium to help the bowels retain the nutriment, were continued. The intense summer heat added greatly to Mr. Garfield's discomfort, and a cooling system was devised in which, by means of an exhaust fan, air entering the sick room was made to pass through Turkish toweling kept wet by a drip of ice water. The resulting drop in room temperature was very satisfactory.

On August 15 swelling of a parotid gland appeared and continued on to eventual suppuration. This complication indicated blood-stream infection and was recognized as a bad omen. At this time it was estimated that the patient had lost weight to the extent of at least seventy-five pounds. He was becoming extremely weary of his situation and begged to be moved. He desired especially to be taken for an ocean cruise. On August 31 the suppurating parotid gland was drained and the relief was great despite the presence of numerous pustules and small boils in the armpits and over the lower back and buttocks. These foci of infection in the skin were opened as they softened.

On September 6, in response to the insistent demands of the patient for a change of air, he was transported by train to Elbernon, New Jersey, and placed in a private residence at the seashore. He was in better spirits following the change, but his doctors felt that the end was only a few days away. On September 8, Surgeon General Barnes, Surgeon Woodward, and Reyburn retired from the case. Dr. Bliss remained in charge and Professors Agnew and Hamilton of New York were retained as consultants. A statement was signed and issued by Drs. Bliss and Hamilton disclaiming any disagreement among the attending doctors or any dissatisfaction with their services on the part of either the President or Mrs. Garfield. On September 19, at ten-thirty P.M., Mr. Garfield complained of sudden, excruciating pain in the heart region, and quickly expired.

An autopsy was performed which, while indicating that the fatal termination of the President's injuries was inevitable, also revealed the most astonishing and humiliating errors of diagnosis by his attending surgeons. It was expected that the wound track would lead the examiners directly to the bullet in the lower right quadrant of the abdomen. But the missile had not entered the abdominal cavity at all. Instead, it had taken a direction at a right angle to the one imagined by the doctors and, after passing through the body of the first lumbar vertebra, had lodged behind the peritoneum at a point well to the left of the spinal column. It lay approximately ten inches from the spot where it was thought to lie. It is remarkable that Dr. Bell's induction-balance device seemed to support the surgeons in their belief that the bullet was in the lower right quadrant of the abdomen.

Dr. Andrew Smith, in his retiring address before the New York Academy of Medicine many years later, told of his part in the autopsy and then described the findings in these words: "The bullet had passed through the body of the first lumbar vertebra in a direction slightly downward and backward and, keeping behind the peritoneum, had lodged at a point just below the level of the left extremity of the pancreas where it became encysted. In its passage it had grazed the splenic artery giving rise to traumatic aneurysm. The rupture of this aneurysm was the immediate cause of death." Dr. D. W. Bliss, who in a spirit of the greatest devotion had spent every night from July 2 to September 19 at the bedside of the wounded President, made this final statement:

"The immediate cause of his death was the spontaneous rupture of a traumatic aneurysm formed on the splenic artery probably as the result of the abrasion of the outer coats of this blood vessel by the bullet at the time of the shooting. This was a complication that could neither be foreseen nor prevented, nor could it have been relieved by any exertion of surgical or medical skill on the part of the surgeons. The proximate cause of death (and one that would inevitably soon have terminated his life even if the bursting of the aneurysm had not taken place) was the profound condition of septic poisoning which existed in the case of the President for a considerable time previous to his death. . . . Finally, while it is difficult and perhaps impossible for anyone to give a dispassionate judgment in a case in which we were all so deeply and personally interested as in that of the President, yet it is my deliberate conviction (as it was of all the surgeons in charge of the case) that the President was mortally wounded when he received the fatal shot. Freely confessing our errors of diagnosis, yet we believe that no different course of treatment could have saved his life. I know that I speak only the truth when I say that no wounded man ever received more devoted service."

Why the surgeons strayed so far afield in their diagnosis is hard to say. Certainly it was not due to a deficiency in the general state of medical knowledge at the time, and it is equally certain that all the elements for an essentially complete clinical diagnosis were present. Exact localization of the bullet, important chiefly for indicating the direction and extent of the wound tract, was not to be expected in the absence of roentgenography (which was first used in 1897). Nor was it of great importance in this instance since a correct interpretation of the clinical signs would have given most of the information sought. The pain in the legs and feet coupled with loss of bowel and bladder control indicated spinal-cord injury almost as plainly as the printed words could do it. Perhaps the fact that the cord symptoms, being due to concussion, disappeared after a week or ten days was confusing. One of the surgeons hinted that the foolish probing of the wound by a certain dominative member of the staff and his assertion that the track led forward to the abdominal cavity misled all the others. Whatever the source of the errors, public confidence in the medical profession at large was dealt a heavy blow.

It may well be asked if the life of President Garfield could have been saved by modern surgery. Under modern surgical conditions, which, of course, are to be had only in properly equipped hospitals, the initial shock and internal hemorrhage would be combated with intravenous injections of plasma or of whole blood combined with the use of such drugs as seemed proper. Nutritional needs would be cared for by feeding carbohydrate and protein substances directly into the blood stream. X-ray examination would be made, to be sure, and without removal of the patient from his bed or room, and the shattered vertebral body and the location of the bullet would be revealed. Operation would discover the wound tract and the source of the internal hemorrhage. Loose fragments of bone and any gross foreign material would be removed and drainage established. Infection would be controlled by penicillin or some other antibiotic. Under this general scheme of treatment in a patient with the President's great stamina, rapid recovery should ensue. Probably the greatest source of danger would be the wound of the splenic artery. It is likely, however, that the initial injury to this vessel was slight and that without severe, prolonged infection of the contiguous wound tract, aneurysm would not have occurred. The answer to the question is, therefore, a qualified—yes.

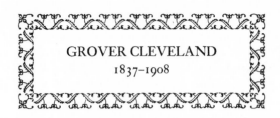

M<small>EDICAL INTEREST</small> in the life of Grover Cleveland centers about a secret operation for cancer performed during his second term in the White House. To appreciate the political significance and dramatic values of the event, we must view it against a backdrop illustrative of the character of the man and the times in which he lived.

The fifth of a family of nine children born to Richard F. and Ann Neal Cleveland, he was christened Stephen Grover. Eventually, however, he dropped the first name and called himself simply Grover Cleveland. The abscission was possibly related to the fact that in the roistering days of his early life as attorney and burgeoning politician in Buffalo, he was known as "Big Steve." It is understandable that he should desire to rid his name of a connotation which might later hinder the advancement of his career.

Cleveland's father was a small-church Presbyterian clergyman, though a graduate of Yale; his mother was the daughter of a Baltimore merchant of Irish extraction. At the time of Grover's birth, the family lived at Caldwell, New Jersey. Within the next fifteen years, however, they moved successively to Fayetteville, New York, Clinton, and Holland Patent. Within a month after taking residence in the last-named town, Richard Cleveland died, apparently of acute appendicitis. Grover was ready to enter college, but the death of his parent forced a change of plans and the sixteen year old lad found employment as teacher in the New

York State Institution for the Blind. The salary was a pittance, but he and his older brother, William, who was head of the Literary Department in the Institution, managed to send a few dollars each month to the family in Holland Patent. At the end of what was perhaps the bleakest year in his entire life Grover decided to seek his fortune in the West. His first stop, at Buffalo to visit an uncle, was his journey's end.

While staying at his uncle's home, Grover was stricken with typhoid and was desperately ill for several weeks. Credit for his recovery was given to a Dr. King, who became greatly attached to the lad and cared for him with the utmost devotion. After he was well again, Grover obtained a job as clerk and copyist for a local law firm. He applied himself assiduously and at the age of twenty-two was admitted to the New York bar. The next year was marked by the beginning of the Civil War and a year after that the conflict was raging furiously, but apparently no martial ardor was kindled in the breast of the young lawyer. Although two of his brothers joined the Union Army in 1861, Grover remained behind seemingly completely absorbed in his profession. When, in 1863, the Conscription Act became effective, he hired a Polish sailor as substitute. It is not recorded that he ever gave a public explanation of why he failed to take up arms in behalf of the Union. It is quite possible that at the beginning of the struggle he felt a strong sympathy for his fellow democrats of the South, and it is known that while his brothers were in the service, he was the principal support of his mother and the younger children. Nevertheless, he recognized the importance of preserving the Union and eventually became a great admirer of President Lincoln.

When Cleveland embarked upon his professional career in Buffalo, the city was a "sink of iniquity," full of saloons, brothels, and gambling houses. Undoubtedly the young lawyer knew the set-up of most of the places, and it is a certainty that he enjoyed an intimate acquaintanceship with the interior of many of the saloons. A coalition machine ruled the city, first under the banner of one party and then under the standard of the other. But no matter which party was in power nominally, the boodle went into the same pockets. Grover, however, took no grist to the corrupt political mill and got no meal from it. Although he loved his beer and convivial companionship, he always denounced with the greatest vehemence every aspect of political chicanery or official dishonesty. Early in his career he attached himself to the large German population of the city whose habits of life suited him exactly. The Germans knew how to work when work was to be done, and they knew how to play when the right to play had been won by honest labor. Moreover, they could be depended upon to support a good friend and good man when the need came.

In 1863 young Cleveland was appointed district attorney of Erie County. Upon expiration of his term, he returned to the private practice of law, having been defeated at the polls when he sought election to the office. In 1870 he was elected sheriff of the county he had served as district attorney. His strict enforcement of the law won him the respect of the better element in the county. At the same time it aroused a minimum of animosity among the saloon and gambling forces, probably because there were no laws to apply to any but the most flagrant cases. In the course of his duties as sheriff, it became necessary to hang two men convicted of first degree murder. As Cleveland disdained to put "so hateful a task" upon a deputy or to hire a professional executioner, he sprang the trap with his own hands. His reputation for official honesty enabled him to win the mayoralty on a reform ticket in 1881. Before his term of office had expired, he resigned to step into the governorship of New York. In 1884 he was nominated for the Presidency on the Democratic ticket, and a bitter contest with Blaine, the Republican nominee, ensued.

At this critical moment revelation of an episode in Cleveland's private life nearly wrecked his prospects for winning the national election. It happened that in September, 1874, an attractive and accomplished widow of thirty-six years, one Maria Halpin, gave birth to a son whom she named Oscar Folsom Cleveland in "honor" of two of her friends, Oscar Folsom and his boon companion, Grover Cleveland. The latter, she charged, was the baby's father. When an opposition newspaper uncovered the affair and Cleveland forthrightly admitted that Mrs. Halpin's allegations could be true and that, on such basis, he had contributed to the support of the child,[1] the effect was truly explosive. The Republican press

[1] The boy was placed in an orphanage, but shortly was adopted by a

came out with gleeful "extras" and the telegraph wires were hot with details of the scandal. Pathetically enough, a large number of influential Republicans, disgusted with the party's choice of a candidate who was openly allied with the lobbyists and spoilsmen, had espoused the cause of Cleveland. A great national meeting was being held by these mugwumps in the University Club Theater in New York on July 22, for mass endorsement of the Democratic nominee. Among those most active in the Cleveland cause were Carl Schurz and George W. Curtis. When the scandalous news broke upon the gathering, the discomfiture of the two was enough to wring a tear from any but the most pachydermatous Republican.

As Curtis groaned and moaned his despair, an unidentified gentleman from Chicago came forth with a cheerful observation which went far to dispel the thickening gloom. "We are told," said the Chicagoan, "that Mr. Blaine has been delinquent in office but blameless in private life, while Mr. Cleveland has been a model of official integrity but culpable in his personal relations. We should, therefore, elect Mr. Cleveland to the public office which he is so well qualified to fill, and remand Mr. Blaine to the private station which he is so admirably fitted to adorn."

Apparently the Chicago genius bespoke the sentiment of the nation, for despite the noisy opposition of the Republican party and the rampant moralists of all parties, Mr. Cleveland won the Presidential contest of 1884. In office he ignored party traditions with respect to the dispensation of patronage and political preferment and thereby antagonized members of Congress and their expectants. To this impolitic behavior many authorities ascribe his failure to be re-elected in the fall of 1888, when he was defeated by the Republican, Benjamin Harrison.

At the expiration of his term, Mr. Cleveland returned to New York and resumed the practice of law. He again entered the political arena in 1892, but because of repeated attacks of gout he was able to make only a few public appearances; despite his inability to wage a personal campaign, he was again elected to the Presidency. Taking office in 1893 in the midst of a financial crisis which

wealthy family of up-state New York. He was given a good education and became a successful and honorable professional man.

his immediate predecessor in the White House had been powerless to avert, President Cleveland soon discovered that his courage and wisdom were about to undergo a supreme test. A powerful silver bloc was seeking, by means of the Sherman Act, to force free coinage of silver and abandonment of the gold standard. Only the fighting opposition of a determined president, it was generally conceded, could steady a vacillating Congress and save the country from the anguish of financial panic. It was known that Vice President Adlai Stevenson either favored the act or, at best, weakly opposed it. Mr. Cleveland accepted the challenge and fought the silverites with every political weapon he could command. *The Commercial and Financial Chronicle* commented moodily, "Mr. Cleveland is about all that stands between this Country and absolute disaster; his death would be a great calamity." *The Nation* said editorially, "A great deal is staked upon the continuance of a single human life." Similar expressions were voiced by the ablest economists and business leaders in the land. Such was the "State of the Union" at the moment when the discovery was made that the President's life was in the gravest danger.

On June 18, 1893, Dr. R. M. O'Reilly, later surgeon general of the United States Army, was called to examine a rough spot on Mr. Cleveland's hard palate. The doctor suspected malignancy and sent a tissue specimen to Dr. William H. Welch, distinguished pathologist at Johns Hopkins, who confirmed the diagnosis. The growth was the size of a quarter of a dollar and extended from the bicuspid teeth on the left to within one-third of an inch of the soft palate. It was found to have invaded the overlying bone of the upper jaw. Dr. O'Reilly advised consultation with Dr. Joseph D. Bryant, eminent surgeon and personal friend of the President. In answer to the latter's inquiry concerning the best procedure, Dr. Bryant replied, "Were it in my mouth, I would have the growth removed at once." That settled the question. Mr. Cleveland instructed Dr. Bryant to go ahead with necessary preparations, but enjoined the greatest secrecy on the part of all concerned. On June 20, Dr. Bryant wrote Secretary of War Lamont that he had enlisted the help of Dr. W. W. Keen, one of the greatest surgeons America has produced, and on June 26 in another message he informed Lamont that on the following Wednesday or Thursday Commodore Benedict's yacht, *Oneida*, would be standing by at Pier A, New York, to receive "our friend who should go aboard on Friday night or at all events early Saturday."

Late in the evening of June 30, the President, Mr. and Mrs. Lamont, and Dr. Bryant arrived in New York and drove openly to the pier. Aboard the yacht the patient and Dr. Bryant found Drs. O'Reilly, Janeway, Hasbrouk, Erdmann, and Keen awaiting them. Hasbrouk was an expert dentist and Erdmann was Bryant's regular assistant. The operation was scheduled for the next day, and Mr. Cleveland was subjected to a careful preoperative examination. The yacht remained anchored in Bellevue Bay all night and the patient slept well without the aid of sedatives.

No one could have been more acutely conscious of his great responsibility than was Dr. Bryant. Fearing that the internes at Bellevue Hospital might recognize members of the medical staff, the Doctor warned the latter to keep out of sight until the *Oneida* was well away from that vicinity. Next morning the saloon was cleared and the yacht began steaming slowly up East River. Mr. Cleveland was propped up in a chair against the ship's mast and administration of the anesthetic was begun. At first nitrous oxide was used; later, when the patient had become unconscious, a switch to ether was made. Satisfactory anesthesia was obtained only after some difficulty. Dr. Hasbrouk then extracted the two left upper bicuspid teeth, following which Dr. Bryant began excision of the growth. He worked rapidly and with great skill, and thirty-one minutes after its beginning, the operation was completed. Most of the left upper jaw was removed, but the orbital plate—the lower wall of the bony cavity containing the eyeball—was left intact. Nor was an external incision necessary. With the fitting of a prosthesis (artificial part) the contour of the face and the characteristic features would be restored. The extensive operation was made necessary by the fact that the surgeons found the normally hollow space in the upper jaw—the maxillary sinus or antrum of Highmore—partially occupied by the gelatinous substance composing the malignant growth. At the moment the growth was thought to be a sarcoma, but Nevins quotes Dr. Erdmann as saying it was later identified as a carcinoma. The wound cavity was packed with gauze to control hemorrhage and the patient was carried to his bed. "What an intense sigh of relief we surgeons breathed when the patient was once more safely in bed, can hardly be imagined," wrote Dr. Keen.

On July 3, two days after the operation, Mr. Cleveland was up and about; on July 5, when the *Oneida* dropped anchor in Buzzards Bay, he was able to walk from the yacht to Gray Gables, his summer home, without undue effort. On July 17 there was a minor operation to remove some suspicious tissue situated at the edge of the wound. Although the President was interviewed by several Cabinet members and by other persons in the weeks between July 23 and September 1 and it was apparent that something was wrong with his mouth, no outsider knew what had occurred. Attorney General Olney was among the first visitors to be received at Gray Gables. He found Mr. Cleveland "changed a good deal in appearance." The President talked little, seemed greatly depressed, and, in Olney's opinion, acted as if he had no hope for recovery. His recuperative and healing powers, however, were remarkably good, and very soon he refused longer to be considered an invalid. On September 1, Dr. Bryant pronounced the operative wound "all healed" and the patient fit to resume his usual activities. Between operations Dr. Kasson C. Gibson of New York had fashioned an artificial jaw of vulcanized rubber which gave the face a perfectly normal appearance and the voice a natural quality.

For nearly two months the operation was kept a complete secret; then on August 29, a reporter known as Holland, whose real name was E. J. Edwards, published in the Philadelphia *Press* a detailed account of the whole affair. Everywhere the story was met with disbelief. It was denied by some who knew the report was true and by others close to the President who had themselves been deceived. L. Clarke Davis wrote the *Press* that the story "has a real basis of a toothache," but if any other, "Mr. Cleveland's closest friends do not know it." He added that he had seen the President frequently since the latter first came to Buzzards Bay, passing hours in his company and in the boat fishing with him, and he had never seen the Chief Executive in better condition physically or mentally. It was reported on good authority that Dr. Bryant blamed Dr. Hasbrouk, the dentist, for the leak and thereafter never would speak or write to him. He even sent Hasbrouk his fee of $250 by messenger. Before the President returned to Washington in September, the odious Sherman Act had been repealed and the purpose of secrecy had been served. But it was not until 1928, when Dr. Keen published a supplement to an earlier article on the surgical operations on President Cleveland, that the exact nature of the surgery and all the circumstances attending it became matters of public knowledge.

With retirement from political life, Mr. Cleveland took up his residence in Princeton, New Jersey, where he immediately became affiliated with Princeton University as occasional lecturer on public affairs. Shortly he was chosen as trustee of the institution. The last years of his life were made happy by the overwhelming tributes of respect and affection accorded him not only by the student body and faculty of the University, but by the American people in general. It was indeed an agreeable disillusionment for the man who, as the doors of the White House closed behind him, thought himself the most hated person in the United States.

Throughout the year 1907, Mr. Cleveland was in failing health, and in the spring of 1908 he took to his bed with arthritis and heart disease. On June 23, the ever sanguine Dr. Bryant reported that he had detected signs of improvement, but the following morning the patient suddenly became unconscious, gasped a few times, and died. The immediate cause of death was believed to have been a blood clot which had formed in the malfunctioning heart and was abruptly transported to the brain by way of the arterial system.

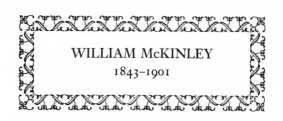

WILLIAM McKINLEY
1843–1901

WILLIAM McKINLEY, twenty-fifth president of the United States, was born in Niles, Trumbull County, Ohio, on January 29, 1843. He was the seventh of a family of nine children. He obtained his early schooling at Poland, Mahoning County, Ohio, and at the age of seventeen entered the junior class of Allegheny College. There he "studied beyond his strength" and quitting college returned to Poland to become a country school teacher. In 1861 he enlisted in the Union Army as a private, and after considerable battle experience he was breveted major "for gallant and meritorious services." After the war he again returned to the town of Poland, this time to occupy himself with the study of law. He completed his preparation at the Albany (New York) School of Law and was admitted to the Ohio bar in 1867. He then took up his residence in Canton and opened a law office in that city. In politics he was a Republican, and he showed himself an able speaker in behalf of the principles of the party. In 1876 he was elected to the United States House of Representatives. In 1891, and again in 1893 he was elected governor of his native state. He was elected to the Presidency of the United States in 1896. During his administration the Spanish-American War was fought and, at its own request, Hawaii was annexed to the United States. In 1900, on the basis of his record, he was re-elected president. His health had not always been good, but there is no record of serious illness at any time.

227

About four o'clock on the afternoon of September 6, 1901, President McKinley was shot twice by a professed anarchist named Leon Czologosz. The shooting had evidently been carefully planned. The President was attending a reception in his honor at the Temple of Music at the Pan-American Exposition in Buffalo, New York. Among those who pressed forward to greet the nation's chief was Czologosz. He concealed a short-barreled thirty-two-caliber revolver in his right hand by covering both weapon and hand with a handkerchief applied in the manner of a surgical bandage. Without removing the handkerchief and with the muzzle of the gun only a few inches from the President's body, Czologosz fired two shots in quick succession. The President, with a look of astonishment, reeled into the arms of a guard named Geary who prevented him from falling to the floor. The wounded man was immediately conveyed to the emergency hospital on the Exposition grounds and placed upon a table in the operating room. As he was being undressed, a bullet fell from his clothing.

Examination disclosed that the first bullet, which was the one lying loose in the clothing, had been deflected, apparently by a button on the President's coat or shirt, and had produced only a superficial wound over the breastbone. The second bullet had entered the upper abdomen slightly to the left of the mid-line. Dr. G. Mc. K. Hall, who was in charge of the hospital at the time, covered the wounds with antiseptic dressings while his assistants, a medical student and a nurse, prepared and administered a hypodermic of one-sixth grain of morphine and one-sixtieth grain of strychnine. Dr. Herman Mynter, a local physician, and Dr. Eugene Wasdin of the United States Marine Hospital, arrived after a few minutes, and seeing that an operation was indicated set about preparing for it. The President asked them to consider him an ordinary patient and to treat his injuries accordingly.

Dr. Matthew D. Mann, a local surgeon of experience and ability, was summoned to perform the operation. Assisting Dr. Mann were Dr. Wallace Lee and Dr. Parmenter. Dr. Eugene Wasdin gave the anesthetic. Under ether narcosis an incision was made parallel to the mid-line of the abdomen and through the wound of entrance. A very heavy layer of subcutaneous fat was encountered. The stomach was exposed and examined. The wound of

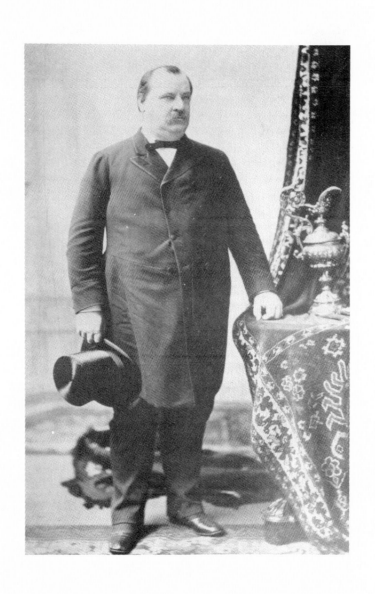

GROVER CLEVELAND

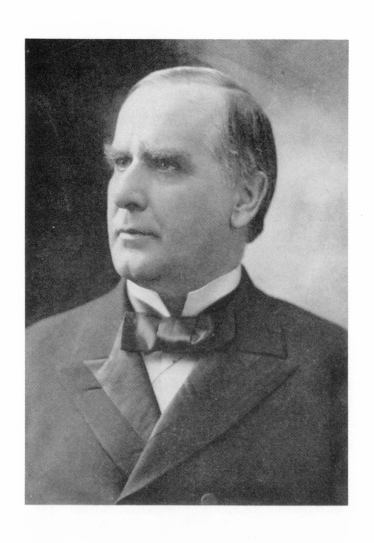

WILLIAM McKINLEY

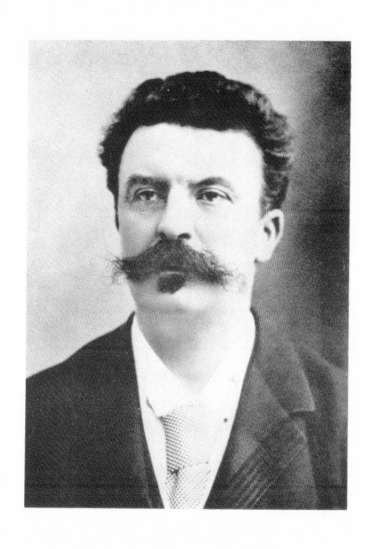

GUY DE MAUPASSANT

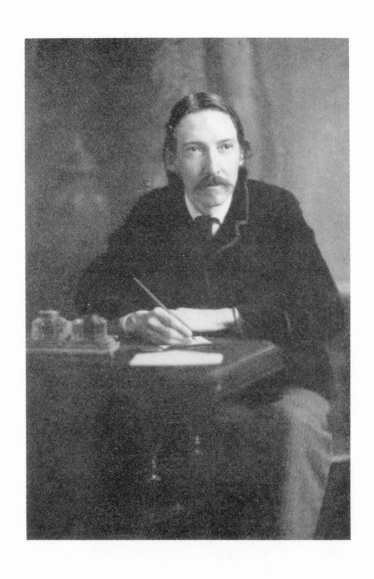

ROBERT LOUIS STEVENSON

the anterior wall was clean cut, and the tissue about it was apparently not much injured. The wound of exit, on the posterior wall, however, was larger and its edges were frayed and infiltrated with blood. There was a small amount of fluid in the stomach. Each wound was encircled with a double row of silk sutures arranged in purse-string fashion and snugly closed. The entire abdominal cavity was washed out with warm normal saline solution. At this juncture, Professor Roswell Park, distinguished surgeon and author of many works on surgery, entered the operating room. Dr. Mann asked him to inspect the operative field and to offer any suggestions he thought pertinent. After a close scrutiny, Dr. Park declared the operation completely satisfactory. No attempt was made to find the bullet, which had apparently entered the posterior abdominal wall. The surgical incision was closed in layers without drainage.

At seven thirty o'clock the President was removed from the hospital by ambulance and taken to a room in the residence of Mr. Milburn, 1168 Delaware Avenue. There he was placed in a hospital bed which had been prepared for him. During the night he was given a hypodermic of morphine. He was slightly nauseated and vomited occasionally. His pulse improved, he voided ninety c.c. of urine, and he retained an enema of normal salt solution.

Second day. The patient slept a good deal and seemed comfortable. Forenoon temperature 102, pulse 110, respiration 24. Much gas was expelled from the bowels. At six-thirty in the evening pulse was 130, temperature 102.5. Examination of the urine was made and the usual findings for a concentrated urine were reported. It was specifically stated that a sugar test was negative. The specific gravity was not given.

Third day. The President slept some. At times he was mentally confused and complained of chilly sensations. The pulse rate was 132, the temperature 102.8. At eight-thirty A.M. his condition was pronounced satisfactory. Dr. Charles McBurney, famous surgeon of New York, arrived, examined the patient, and consulted with Dr. Mann and others who were in attendance. At nine-thirty P.M., the President's pulse was 130, temperature 101.6. He voided 460 c.c. of urine during the day. Examination of the voided specimen revealed a trace of albumin as the only significant finding. No sugar was found. The specific gravity was 1.026.

Fourth day. At six A.M., the pulse rate was 120, temperature 101, and respiration 28. At nine-thirty P.M., the pulse was 112, temperature 101, respiration 27. Codeine was substituted for morphine. Sips of hot water were permitted and nutritive enemas given. Again a complete urinary examination was made. There remained a trace of albumin, but no sugar was found. The specific gravity was 1.026.

Fifth day. It was announced that Mr. McKinley had spent the most comfortable night yet. He was free of pain and his mood was cheerful. Nutritive enemas were continued. The bowels moved twice during the day. A little slough was noticed at the edges of the surgical incision and, to permit free drainage, four stitches were removed from the skin. Immediately the wound gaped down to the muscle layer. It was irrigated with hydrogen dioxide.

Sixth day. The morning condition was reported excellent. The stomach tolerated beef juice, which was taken with great relish. The morning pulse was 116, the temperature 100.2. A blood count was made and the results were: Leucocytes 6,752, red-blood count 3,920,000 per cu. m.m. The patient was cheerful and comfortable. The wound looked clean. 750 c.c. of urine were voided in twenty-four hours. Examination of a specimen was made. Findings were noted with respect to quantity, color, reaction, albumin, indican, phosphates, and sulfates. No mention was made of a test for sugar. The specific gravity was 1.027.

There was much public clamor for an X-ray examination to determine the location of the bullet. As such an examination would involve moving the patient and as the missile was deemed to have already done all the mischief of which it was capable, the doctors announced that an X-ray examination was considered neither necessary nor advisable.

Seventh day. The President slept well during the night and felt well in the morning. He seemed to be in excellent condition. The bowels moved freely, the tongue was clean, and the appetite was increasing. There was no tenderness in the abdomen and the patient was able to turn easily and to lie on either side. He was in good spirits and his pulse was strong though rapid. Dr. McBurney, satisfied with the progress of the case, returned to New York. At eight-thirty P.M. the condition was not quite so favorable as during the day. The pulse was 128, the temperature 100.2. Calomel was administrated at seven P.M. and followed by castor oil two hours later. Then a high enema of oxgall was given. A large, dark stool resulted, but the procedure seemed to tire the patient. Again a urinary examination, complete except for a sugar test, was reported. The specific gravity was 1.025.

Eighth day. At two-fifty A.M. the pulse was 126, respiration 30, and the temperature 100. The President seemed very sick, arousing the gravest apprehension. At six-thirty P.M. his condition appeared critical. Despite vigorous stimulation, the pulse was steadily growing weaker. At nine-thirty P.M., the heart sounds were feeble and the patient was unconscious. Oxygen was administered. Again a urinary examination was reported without mention of a test for sugar. The specific gravity was 1.023.

Ninth day, September 14. It was announced that President McKinley had expired at two-fifteen A.M. Before the body was removed from the Milburn home, an autopsy was done by Dr. Harvey R. Gaylor, pathologist, and Dr. Herman G. Matzinger, bacteriologist, of the New York State Pathological Laboratories. Before their official report was made, however, the doctors who had attended President McKinley and witnessed the autopsy issued the following statement setting forth the essential findings:

> The bullet which struck over the breast-bone did not pass through the skin and did little harm. The other bullet passed through both walls of the stomach near its lower border. Both holes were found to be perfectly closed by the stitches but the tissue around each hole had become gangrenous. After passing through the stomach the bullet passed into the back wall of the abdomen hitting and tearing the upper end of the kidney. This portion of the bullet track was also gangrenous, the gangrene involving the pancreas. The bullet has not yet been found. There was no sign of peritonitis or disease of other organs. The heart walls were very thin. There was no evidence of any attempt at repair on the part of nature, and

death resulted from the gangrene which affected the stomach around the bullet wounds as well as the tissues around the further course of the bullet. Death was unavoidable by any surgical or medical treatment and was the direct result of the bullet wound.

After the lapse of a number of days, Dr. Gaylord made public a detailed account of the course of the fatal bullet and the organs involved. Of special interest is his description of the damaged pancreas. Said he,

> The necrotic cavity which connects the wound on the posterior wall of the stomach and the opening adjacent to the kidney capsule is walled off by the mesocolon and is found to involve an area of the pancreas approximately 45 m.m. in diameter and extending halfway through the organ. This organ at its center forms part of the necrotic cavity. Through its body are found numerous minute hemorrhages and areas of gray softening the size of a pea or smaller. These are less frequent in the head portion of the pancreas.[1]

It is regrettable that no microscopic examination of the pancreas was reported, and it seems probable that none was made since Dr. Gaylord appended the remark, "Embarrassment arose in the objection to our removing sufficient portions of the tissues for examination." With respect to the search for the fatal missile, Dr. Gaylord had this to say: "We were requested to desist seeking for the bullet and to terminate the autopsy." From what source request for termination of the autopsy came is not made clear.

The failure of the President's wounds to heal and the inability of his doctors to find a satisfactory explanation for the apparent loss of healing power occasioned considerable speculation among both the laity and the members of the medical profession at large. One theory widely exploited by the press proposed that Czologosz had used bullets poisoned by some chemical substance or by the germs of disease. Curare, an arrow poison used by certain South American Indians was mentioned, but when it was stated au-

[1] The islands of Langerhans are found principally in the distal half (tail) of the pancreas.

thoritatively that neither curare nor any other poison known to science could produce either the symptoms or the lesions observed in Mr. McKinley's case, the theory of chemical or drug poisoning quickly evaporated. A similar fate befell the conjecture that infected bullets were used, after Dr. Herman Matzinger, state bacteriologist, reported that cultures made from the bullets remaining in the cylinder of the revolver after the shooting showed no unusual organisms.

Failure of wounds to heal is especially characteristic of loss of essential pancreatic function, while prostration and rapid death are characteristic of necrosis of the organ. The clinical course of President McKinley's case and the findings reported by the pathologist who conducted the autopsy strongly indicate that death was due to a damaged pancreas. The operation was well done and the fatal outcome cannot, in reason, be attributed to faulty surgery in the aspects of either commission or omission. President McKinley, unlike the rugged Garfield, was not a first-class surgical risk in the beginning. He was fat, his heart walls "were very thin," and he was well along in the fifty-ninth year of his life. Pancreatic surgery was unknown in those days and had the organ been successfully removed, the patient would have succumbed to diabetes very quickly. Even under modern surgical conditions the final outcome would probably have been the same.

It is extraordinary that out of a total of six urine examinations, sugar tests were reported for the first three only. It is inconceivable that examination for sugar was not made in the final three, for even in those days the sugar test was recognized as one of the two most important tests in routine urinalysis. *A specific gravity of 1.027 in a twenty-four-hour total of 750 c.c. of urine* certainly suggests a fairly heavy sugar content, though it is not absolute proof of the presence of sugar in any amount. Even though the patient was taking little nourishment, extensive destruction of the pancreatic islands of Langerhans, the normal source of insulin, would cause the appearance of sugar in the urine.

If sugar was detected in any of the examinations, then, in simple honesty, the fact should have been recorded. Since the attending surgeons were men of unquestioned honor and integrity, we must assume that the omission of the sugar tests somehow escaped their notice. At that time a relationship between disturbed pancreatic function and *diabetes mellitus* was beginning to be suspected. If, as the evidence indicates, the President of the United States actually developed diabetes in association with injury to the pancreas and the fact had been publicized, both impetus and direction would have been given to a line of research which might have been fruitful indeed.[2] It is entirely conceivable that the discovery of insulin might have been accomplished well before 1921 when Banting and Best prepared pancreatic extracts which were found to contain the active principle known thereafter as insulin. In this connection a letter from Dr. R. B. Barrow of Wilmerding, Pennsylvania, published in *American Medicine* a few days after the President's death but before the autopsy findings were made public, deserves respectful attention. Dr. Barrow wrote:

> It would be of interest to know if an examination of President McKinley's urine showed the presence of sugar previous to and after he was shot. I take it that the gangrene which occurred was the kind due to the malnutrition which accompanies diabetes mellitus and not to a poisoned bullet. It seems to me that if the final course of the bullet and its exact location had been ascertained this case might have thrown some light upon the subject of the causal relationship which exists between diseases of the pancreas, lesions of the nervous system, and diabetes.

To have served in death as importantly as he served in life might have been the unique privilege of President McKinley.

[2] About half a dozen cases of diabetes following violence to the pancreas have been recorded. See the *Journal of the American Medical Association,* Vol. 147, No. 15, p. 1507.

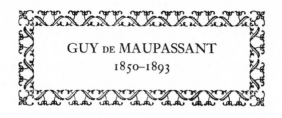

GUY DE MAUPASSANT
1850–1893

G UY DE MAUPASSANT, "master of the short story,"
was of Norman extraction and spent the first few years of his life
in the vicinity of Rouen. In early manhood he became a clerk in
the Ministry of Marine in Paris, a position which he neglected
earnestly in favor of boating on the Seine or experimenting with
the art of short-story writing. His literary efforts attracted the
attention of Gustave Flaubert, who encouraged him to cultivate
the faculty of minute observation as a prerequisite to accuracy of
statement and vividness of description.

Although his writings are tinctured with a certain morbid-
ness, they do not, in general, reflect the depravity of character
which is said to have marred his private life. He has been called
"a faun with sensual features and a Cro-Magnon jaw; the sort of
man who would brazenly take leave of his companions on the
street or on the River in order to visit a bagnio or waterside
brothel." Also, "a foul mouthed offensive individual" totally destitute of a sense of decency.

As early as 1884, Maupassant revealed evidences of mental
disquietude when he wrote his story, "*Lui*," in which he confesses
a fear "of the walls, of the furniture, of the familiar objects which
seem to me to assume a kind of animal life. Above all I fear the
horrible confusion of my thought, of my reason escaping, en-
tangled and scattered by an invisible and mysterious anguish."

235

And in "*Le Horla*," written in 1887, he records strange fears un-doubtedly personal and genuine, which grow on him despite his reason, which tells him that they are without basis in fact. He con-cludes rightly that some disturbance has arisen in his brain; that he has thoughts which no rational being should have. But the mys-terious pressure is unrelenting, pushing him ever nearer the border of insanity until he cries in despair, "I am lost! Somebody possesses my soul and dominates it. Somebody orders all my acts, all my movements, all my thoughts. I am no longer anything in myself, nothing except an enslaved and terrified spectator of all the things I do."

He plans to kill and destroy the thing which has mastered him, but concludes despondently that it is something invisible and im-palpable and therefore unassailable. He chances to read a news account of a fearful madness which has attacked the populace in the province of São Paulo, Brazil, and he is reminded instantly of a fine three-masted Brazilian ship which he had admired a few months before as it passed by his window on its way up the Seine. He concludes that the Being was on board the ship and that it sprang from the ship to the land to take possession of his brain.

Two years after he had written "*Le Horla*," Maupassant was obviously insane, though he seems not to have been confined in an asylum until 1892 following an attempt at suicide. The invisible thing which had taken possession of his brain was visible under a microscope, as was demonstrated by the Japanese pathologist, Noguchi, who found it in the brain of another victim in the year 1913. It was the *Treponema pallidum*, the causative organism of syphilis.

It is probable that Maupassant acquired his syphilis in his late youth or early maturity and that after a few months it became asymptomatic only to emerge, after a dozen years or more, as paretic neuro-spyhilis, a late manifestation of the disease charac-terized histologically by degenerative changes in the cells of the cerebral cortex and symptomatically by progressive dementia. Un-til recent times paretic dementia invariably came to a fatal termina-tion within from three to ten years, the great majority of its vic-tims dying before the end of the fifth year. Remissions lasting as long as six months occasionally occurred. Maupassant seemed better and worse by turns over a period of several years before the final descensus.

In about 15 per cent of the cases of paretic dementia a classic syndrome occurs in which the afflicted one experiences delusions of grandeur, living in a state of constant elation, imagining himself to be a person of inexhaustible wealth and great influence. There are several other symptomatic types in which the patient is not so fortunate. Maupassant's case belonged to the most wretched of these. His mental breakdown was attended by "migrane, melancholia, obsessions, perversions, hallucinations, and outbreaks of violent, ill-tempered behavior." He died in Paris in 1893 under the most miserable circumstances.

A good deal has been written on the "neurotic heredity" of Maupassant and its relationship to his insanity. Such imputations of inherited affliction are often doubly unjust; they may falsely accuse innocent progenitors and at the same time cast unwarranted reflection upon the initiative of younger generations who are quite capable of seeking out and acquiring their own diseases.

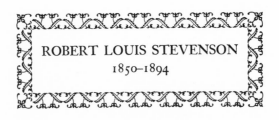

ROBERT LOUIS STEVENSON
1850–1894

P ROBABLY NO AUTHOR in all the world of English literature is better loved than Robert Louis Stevenson. The product of his pen is read with keen enjoyment; his lifelong struggle against illness is recalled with deep compassion.

Stevenson was born and reared in Edinburgh, Scotland. Through the first year of his life he seemed a normal, healthy infant. About the middle of his second year, however, he turned sickly and never again attained his original vigor. It is generally believed that he certainly would have perished but for the ministrations of his nurse, Alison Cunningham, who cared for him with the utmost devotion.

It is a matter of common knowledge that Stevenson suffered from pulmonary tuberculosis. The source of his contagion, however, seems not generally known, nor the fact that his death was due to a cause probably unrelated to his tuberculosis.

Dr. Lewis J. Moorman, in his book entitled *Tuberculosis and Genius*, writes of Stevenson: "At about 18 months of age there was an obvious change in his physical condition. We find in his own writings references to his health which carry us back to the period of early childhood. 'My health principally chronicles itself by the terrible long nights. I lay awake troubled continually with a hacking exhausting cough and praying for sleep or morning from the bottom of my shaken little body.' Or, being carried by the nurse and shown the lighted windows across the dark belt of gardens 'where also, we told each other, there might be sick little boys and their nurses waiting like us for the morning.' It was at this time in Stevenson's life that his mother was making the round of health resorts in an attempt to find what she might consider a suitable climate for her own pulmonary condition."

Dr. Moorman's account thus identifies for us a "contact" which, known or unknown, indispensably precedes the inception of every case of pulmonary tuberculosis. It is a fair conclusion that Stevenson acquired the disease from his mother while yet in his infancy.

Like his mother, Robert Louis traveled far and wide in search of health. He found that his condition improved in southern France and deteriorated in the British Isles. In 1879, however, he made a sentimental journey to California in pursuit of an American lady, Mrs. Fanny Van de Grift Osbourne, whom he had met at Fontaine-bleau and for whom he had developed an ardent affection. From September to December he lived at Monterey, whence he moved to San Francisco where for three months he lived in a workman's lodging-house. He was short of funds, and his health and strength were at a low ebb when some months later he was fortunately married to Mrs. Osbourne, who affectionately dedicated herself and her means to the welfare of her husband. For a time they lived in a deserted mining camp in the California Coast Range, after which they returned to England. Soon it became apparent that Stevenson's health was again in a decline, so they took up their residence for the winter at Davos, Switzerland, going to South France in the spring. But Robert Louis loved his parents and Britain; and, after a residence of two years in the French Mediterranean area, he and his wife again returned to England where he nearly died of hemorrhages. He lay abed for months; at times he was not even permitted to speak aloud. In October, 1887, he was able to make the trip to Saranac Lake, in the New York Adirondacks, where he remained until the following April under the care of the famous Dr. Trudeau. Trudeau was a practical man of science, the exact antithesis of the dreamy-minded Stevenson and his world of fanci-ful unreality. Although their relations were quite friendly, neither was able to share the interests of the other. The Doctor left this note on R.L.S.: "He did not care to go to the sanatorium with me to see the laboratory because to him these were unpleasant things." And, "To a temperament like Stevenson's who shrank from the cruel and inexorable facts of life—disease, suffering, and death—which were a part of my daily existence, I represented, I am afraid, not a very cheerful, inspiring companion."

In June, 1888, Stevenson, with his wife and his mother, left San Francisco on a cruise of the South Pacific which resulted, eventually, in his taking up his permanent abode on the island of Upola, Samoa, in 1891. There for three years he enjoyed the best health he had known since his early days in the south of France.

Considering his state of continuous ill health, it seems a wonder that Stevenson was able to accomplish any work at all. In a letter to George Meredith in 1893 he reveals how his *furor scribendi* drove him on against all reason. "For fourteen years," he wrote, "I have not had a day's real health. I have wakened sick and gone to bed weary and I have done my work unflinchingly. I have written in bed and written out of it, written in hemorrhages, written in sickness, written torn by coughing, written when my head swam for weakness, and for so long, it seems to me, I have won my wager and recovered my glove. I am better now; have been, rightly speaking, since first I came to the Pacific; and still few are the days when I am not in some physical distress. And the battle goes on—ill or well is a trifle—so it goes. I was made for a contest and the Powers have so willed it that my battlefield should be this dingy, inglorious one of the bed and the physic bottle."

The end, which came quickly and unexpectedly on December 3, 1894, as he was making a salad for the evening meal, is described circumstantially by Osbourne, one of Stevenson's biographers: "He was helping his wife on the veranda and gaily talking when suddenly he put both hands to his head and cried out, 'What's that?' Then he asked quickly, 'Do I look strange?' Even as he did so he fell on his knees beside her." Two hours later he died without having regained consciousness after the instant of collapse. Quite obviously the immediate cause of death was cerebral hemorrhage.

Some aspects of Stevenson's illnesses seem worthy of comment. First of all, it may be stated that the extreme chronicity of his pulmonary infection indicates fairly good resistance to the disease. His frequent attacks of hemorrhage in his adult years may be taken as proof that cavity formation had occurred in the lung substance. Taken before the stage of cavitation, progress of the disease might very well have been arrested by such simple measures as prolonged physical and mental rest, adequate diet, and cheerful surroundings. A pleasant climate might have made the regimen less onerous; otherwise it would have been of little importance.

Modern management of Stevenson's case would, ideally, have revealed the presence of tuberculosis in the mother prior to birth of the infant. Immediately after delivery the child would have been taken from the mother, with her consent, and kept apart from her until either she was no longer a source of contagion or he had reached an age when limited guarded association might be safely permissible.

Some physicians would have advised vaccination with the Calmette-Guerin bacillus, an attenuated strain of tubercle bacillus which is being used increasingly for the protective inoculation of newborn infants.

Taken too late for preventive treatment, active treatment could, if necessary, have added certain valuable surgical procedures to the hygienic and immunization measures already mentioned. Such surgical procedures are designed to put the diseased lung at rest and are therefore fully applicable in instances where but one of the lungs is seriously affected. Of first importance is "collapse therapy," usually in the form of artificial pneumothorax, in which a layer of air or other gas is interposed between the lung and the chest wall to form a sort of pneumatic splint for the diseased lung. In desperate cases where pleuritic adhesions make simple collapse impossible, the desideratum may be achieved by the operation of thoracoplasty in which a number of ribs are removed, permitting the diseased lung and the chest wall to collapse en masse. As may be imagined, the operation of thoracoplasty results in considerable deformity, but it may not only save life; it may also restore health and the capacity for moderate physical activity.

Another surgical measure sometimes employed in lieu of thoracoplasty consists of exposure and deliberate traumatization of the phrenic nerve controlling movement of the diaphragm on the affected side. An incision is made in the appropriate part of the neck in order to expose the nerve which is then crushed, resulting in temporary paralysis of that half of the diaphragm supplied by the traumatized nerve. The result is a stoppage of involuntary and a limitation of voluntary respiratory movement on that side of the chest. A certain amount of retraction of the lung ensues in its long axis, but by no means enough to deserve the term "collapse." The operational hazard is practically nil, but generally speaking the results have not been very good. Recently, however, the value of the procedure has been greatly enhanced by its employment as an adjunct to pneumo-peritoneum. In this stratagem, air or inert gas is injected into the peritoneal cavity to distend the abdomen to the limit of patient tolerance. The half of the diaphragm which has been prepared by phrenic nerve paralysis is usually pushed upward several inches at its dome and the adjacent lung undergoes a considerable degree of collapse.

The usefulness of the several operative procedures just described is dependent upon the achievement and maintenance of collapse and immobilization of the damaged lung. In cases where both lungs are extensively involved in the disease process, full utilization of collapse therapy is, of course, impossible.

There is abundant evidence that the antibiotic substance, streptomycin, has power to retard the growth of the tubercle bacillus in living tissue. A lesser effect has been obtained with certain synthetic drugs. It is not too much to hope that the combination of hygiene, vaccination, and specific anti-tuberculosis drugs will, within the next two generations, virtually eliminate this historic destroyer of mankind.

Stevenson's death by cerebral hemorrhage is somewhat surprising in that it suggests antecedent high blood pressure, a condition not commonly associated with active tuberculosis. It must not be inferred, however, that high blood pressure is a *sine qua non* for cerebral vascular disease, since cerebral hemorrhage does sometimes occur in persons believed never to have had high blood pressure. Into which of the two categories Stevenson's case belongs can never be known since instruments for the measurement of blood pressure were unknown to the physicians of his time.

To what extent Stevenson's ailments influenced his manner

of thinking is conjectural. Do his highly imaginative writings represent a mechanism of escape from the distressing immobility of chronic ill health? Were his mental faculties unduly activated by the toxins of his tuberculosis? Dr. Moorman says, ". . . we may well wonder whether or not early intimate contact with his tuberculous mother may have initiated an infection which, directly or indirectly, influenced the trend of his exceptional mind. Granting that from a scientific standpoint this is purely speculative, we can say without fear of contradiction that his early social isolation on account of his physical frailty did materially influence his mental development."

Stevenson did considerable traveling by boat and invariably found exhiliration and improved health in sea voyages. It is not recorded, however, that he was a hunter, except in pursuit of health, and the simple beauty of the "Requiem" must not be impaired by a strictly literal interpretation of the second stanza:

> Under the wide and starry sky
> Dig the grave and let me lie.
> Glad did I live and gladly die,
> And I laid me down with a will.
>
> This be the verse you grave for me:
> *Here he lies where he longed to be;*
> *Home is the sailor, home from the sea,*
> *And the hunter home from the hill.*

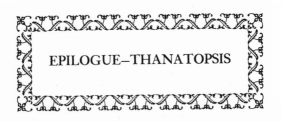

EPILOGUE–THANATOPSIS

THE fact of death is undeniable and inalterable. From the purely evolutionist point of view it is well that death cannot be abolished. We must not be dispirited by the gloomy eloquence of men like Bertrand Russell, who wrote, "Brief and powerless is man's life; on him and all his race the slow sure doom falls pitiless and dark."

In general, mankind fears death less than the painful associations of death. For those who are conscious of the recent advances which have been made in the development of pain-preventing drugs, death has largely lost its greatest terror. Better yet, perhaps, lifesaving surgical procedures which otherwise might be more dreadful than death can now be faced with equanimity. Remembering that the dying do not fear to die and only the fear of death is terrible, each of us may condition himself for acceptance of the end of life as we know it in this world.

In the first pages of this volume are recounted the principal events observed in the demise of an ancient and noble philosopher who won the victory over death; for whether by philosophy, creed, or simple resignation, he who has conquered the fear of death has, in a humanistic sense, conquered death itself.

REFERENCES AND SOURCES

While the thirty-three persons whose medical histories are discussed are listed chronologically in the text, for convenience they are listed alphabetically here.

BUDDHA

Alvarez, Walter C. *Introduction to Gastroenterology.* 4th ed. New York, Paul B. Hoeber, Inc., 1948.

Beck, L. Adams. *Oriental Philosophy.* New York, Cosmopolitan Book Corporation, 1931.

Cecil, Russell L. *A Textbook of Medicine.* 8th ed. Philadelphia, W. B. Saunders Company, 1951.

Herold, A. Ferdinand. *The Life of Buddha.* Trans. from the French by Paul A. Blum. New York, Albert and Charles Boni, 1927.

Stoll, Henry F. "An Early Case of Coronary Thrombosis Not Hitherto Reported," *American Heart Journal,* Vol. IX, No. 3 (February, 1934).

Thomas, Edward J. *The Life of Buddha: Its Legend and History.* New York, Alfred A. Knopf, 1927.

LORD BYRON

"Byron's Lameness and Death," editorial in *British Medical Journal,* Vol. I (April 19, 1924), 719.

Cecil, Russell L. *A Textbook of Medicine.* 8th ed. Philadelphia, W. B. Saunders Company, 1951.

"The Centenary of Byron's Death," *British Medical Journal,* Vol. I (April 19, 1924), 724.

Concise Dictionary of National Biography. London, Oxford University Press, 1930.

Kemble, James. *Idols and Invalids*. Garden City, Doubleday, Doran and Company, 1936.

Lewin, Philip. *The Foot and Ankle*. Philadelphia, Lea and Febiger, 1947.

Maurois, André. *Byron*. New York, D. Appleton and Company, 1930.

Russell, Paul F., Luther S. West, and Reginald D. Manwell. *Practical Malariology*. 1st ed. Philadelphia, W. B. Saunders Company, 1946.

CATHERINE THE GREAT

Anthony, Katharine. *Catherine the Great*. New York, Garden City Publishing Company, 1925.

————. *Memoirs of Catherine the Great*. New York, Alfred A. Knopf, 1927.

Gribble, Francis. *The Comedy of Catherine the Great*. London, Eveleigh Nash, 1912.

Hodgetts, E. A. Brayley. *The Life of Catherine the Great of Russia*. New York, Brentano's, 1914.

Kaus, Gina. *Catherine*. Trans. by June Head. New York, Viking Press, Inc., 1935.

BENVENUTO CELLINI

Becker, S. William, and Maximilian E. Obermayer. *Modern Dermatology and Syphilology*. Philadelphia, J. B. Lippincott Company, 1947.

Cecil, Russell L. *A Textbook of Medicine*. 8th ed. Philadelphia, W. B. Saunders Company, 1951.

Cellini, Benvenuto. *Autobiography*. Trans. by John Addington Symonds. New York, Garden City Publishing Company, 1927.

————. *Memoirs*. Trans. by Anne MacDonell. New York, E. P. Dutton and Company, 1907.

Symonds, J. A. *Renaissance in Italy*. 7 vols. New York, Charles Scribner's Sons, 1907–1908.

CHARLEMAGNE

Baker, G. P. *Charlemagne*. New York, Dodd, Mead and Company, 1932.

Einhard (Eginhard). "Life of the Emperor Charles" (trans. from the Latin by E. S. Turner), in *Great Short Biographies of Ancient Times*, compiled by Barrett H. Clark. New York, Albert and Charles Boni, 1932.

Russell, Charles E. *Charlemagne, First of the Moderns*. Boston, Houghton Mifflin Company, 1930.

Robinson, James Harvey. *Mediaeval and Modern Times*. New York, Ginn and Company, 1919.

GROVER CLEVELAND

Erdman, John F. Personal communication to the author, April 4, 1949.

Gilder, R. W. *Grover Cleveland*. New York, The Century Company, 1910.

Keen, W. W. *The Surgical Operations on President Cleveland, and Six Other Papers of Reminiscences*. Philadelphia, J. B. Lippincott Company, 1928.

Lynch, Denis Tilden. *Grover Cleveland*. New York, Horace Liveright, Inc., 1932.

McElroy, Robert. *Grover Cleveland*. 2 vols. New York, Harper and Brothers, 1923.

Nevins, Allan. *Grover Cleveland*. New York, Dodd, Mead and Company, 1933.

Parker, George F. "Grover Cleveland's Life in Princeton," *The Saturday Evening Post*, November 10, 1923.

Seelig, M. G. "The Operation on Grover Cleveland," *Surgery, Gynecology, and Obstetrics*, Vol. LXXXV, No. 3 (September, 1947), 373-76.

CHRISTOPHER COLUMBUS

Book Notices, *Journal of the American Medical Association*, Vol. CIX, No. 2 (July 10, 1937).

Irving, Washington. *A History of the Life and Voyages of Christopher Columbus*. New York and London, G. P. Putnam's Sons, n.d.

Lamartine, Alphonse de. "Columbus," in *Great Short Biographies of Ancient Times*, compiled by Barrett H. Clark. New York, Albert and Charles Boni, 1932.

Morison, Samuel Eliot. *Admiral of the Ocean Sea.* 2 vols. Boston, Little, Brown and Company, 1942.

Ybarra, A. M. Ferdinand de. "Medical History of Christopher Columbus," *Journal of the American Medical Association*, Vol. XXII (1894), 647–54.

CHARLES DARWIN

Alvarez, Walter C. "Gastroenterology," *Journal of the American Medical Association*, Vol. CXXXII (December 21, 1946), 970.
——. *Nervousness, Indigestion, and Pain.* New York, Paul B. Hoeber, Inc., 1903.

Darwin, Charles. *Life and Letters.* Ed. by Francis Darwin. New York, D. Appleton and Company, 1887.
——. *More Letters.* Ed. by Francis Darwin. New York, D. Appleton and Company, 1903.

Johnson, W. W. "The Ill-Health of Charles Darwin, Its Nature and Its Relation to His Work," *Transactions* of the Medical Society of the District of Columbia, Vol. VI (1902), 7–11.

West, Geoffrey. *Charles Darwin.* New Haven, Yale University Press, 1938.

Winans, Henry M. "Indigestion, a Problem of Office Practice," *American Practitioner*, Vol. II, No. 9 (May, 1948), 56–57.

Wolf, Stewart and Harold G. "Life Situations, Emotions, and Gastric Function," *American Practitioner*, Vol. III, No. 1 (September, 1948), 1–14.

FREDERICK THE GREAT

Carlyle, Thomas. *History of Friedrich the Second, Called Frederick the Great.* 6 vols. New York, Harper and Brothers, 1871.

Goldsmith, Margaret. *Frederick the Great.* New York, Albert and Charles Boni, 1930.

Hegemann, Werner. *Frederick the Great.* Trans. by Winifred Ray. New York, Alfred A. Knopf, 1929.

Lang, Will. "The Case of the Distinguished Corpses," *Life* magazine, March 6, 1950.

Meine, Franklin J., and H. Gaylord Warren. *Great Leaders.* Chicago, University of Knowledge, Inc., 1938.

White, Paul Dudley. *Heart Disease.* 2nd ed. New York, The Macmillan Company, 1937.

FREDERICK III OF PRUSSIA

Ficarra, Bernard J. "Eleven Famous Autopsies in History," *Annals of Medical History*, 3 Ser., Vol. IV (November, 1942), 504–20.

Ludwig, Emil. *Kaiser Wilhelm II*. New York, G. P. Putnam's Sons, 1928.

"Medical Protocol Concerning the Result of the Examination of the Body of His Majesty, the late Emperor and King, Frederick III,'" *British Medical Journal*, July 21, 1888, p. 141.

Stevenson, R. Scott. *Morrell Mackenzie*. New York, Henry Schuman, 1947.

Virchow, Prof. Rudolph. "*Bericht uber der von Dr. Mackenzie extirpirten Theile aus dem Kehlkopfe Seiner K. K. Hoheit, des Kronprinzen*," *Berliner Klinische Wochenschrift*, No. 25 (June 20, 1887).

JAMES A. GARFIELD

Dale, Emma J. "Memories." MS in the library of the Nebraska State Historical Society. 1936.

Editorial, *Journal of the American Medical Association*, Vol. XXXVII (September 21, 1901), 779.

Ficarra, Bernard J. "Eleven Famous Autopsies in History," *Annals of Medical History*, 3 Ser., Vol. IV (November, 1942), 515–16.

Reyburn, Robert. "Clinical History of the Case of President James Abram Garfield," *Journal of the American Medical Association*, Vol. XXII (March 24–May 5, 1894).

———. "The Case of President James A. Garfield" [an abstract of "The Clinical History . . ." listed above], *American Medicine*, Vol. IX (January 21, 1905).

Smith, Andrew H. "President Garfield at Elbernon," *American Medicine*, Vol. IX (January 21, 1905), 118–20.

Smith, Theodore Clark. *Life and Letters of James Abram Garfield*. New Haven, Yale University Press, 1925.

GEORGE III

Adams, James Truslow. *Building the British Empire*. New York, Charles Scribner's Sons, 1938.

Bett, Walter R. "George III," The *British Medical Journal*, Vol. II (September 24, 1938), 664.

Diller, Theodore. *Transactions* of the American Neurological Association, 67th Annual Meeting, June, 1941, p. 229.

May, T. E. "George III," in *New Larned History*, IV, 2791–92. 12 vols. Springfield, Mass., C. A. Nichols Publishing Company, 1923.

Overholser, Winfred. "Famous Madcaps of History," *Bulletin 43*, Chicago Medical Society (1943), 314–18.

EDWARD GIBBON

Cambridge History of English Literature, X. New York, G. P. Putnam's Sons, 1913.

Gibbon, Edward. *Memoirs of My Life and Writings* in Vol. I of 6 vol. ed. of *The Decline and Fall of the Roman Empire*. New York, Harper and Brothers, 1905.

Sheffield, Lord. "Last Illness and Death of Gibbon," in Vol. I of above.

Thorex, Max. *Modern Surgical Technique*. 3 vols. Philadelphia, J. B. Lippincott, 1938. Vol. III, 1967–72.

Watson, Leigh F. *Hernia*. St. Louis, C. V. Mosby Company, 1938.

HENRY VIII

Appleby, L. H. "The Medical Life of Henry the Eighth," *Bulletin* of the Vancouver Medical Association, Vol. X (March, 1934), 87–101.

Davidson, Israel. "Fetal Erythroblastosis," *Journal of the American Medical Association*, Vol. CXXVII, No. 11 (March 17, 1945).

Editorial, *Journal of the American Medical Association*, Vol. CXV (June 17, 1944), 495.

Fitzpatrick, Benedict. *Frail Anne Boleyn*. New York, Dial Press, 1931.

Flugel, I. C. "On the Character and Married Life of Henry VIII," *International Journal of Psychoanalysis*, Vol. I (1920), 24–55.

Hackett, Francis. *Henry the Eighth*. New York, H. Liveright, 1920.

Hume, David. *The Wives of Henry VIII.* 4th ed. London, Eveleigh Nash and Grayson, n.d.

Kemble, J. "Henry VIII, a Psychological Survey and a Surgical Explanation," *Annals of Medical History,* new ser., Vol. III (November, 1931), 619–25.

———. *Idols and Invalids.* Garden City, Doubleday, Doran and Company, 1936.

Macomber, D. "Lowered Fertility in the Male," *Journal of the American Medical Association,* Vol. LXXXV (November 21, 1925), 1603–1605.

Morison, Samuel Eliot. *Admiral of the Ocean Sea.* 2 vols. Boston, Little, Brown and Company, 1942.

Stokes, John H., Herman Beerman, and Norman Ingraham, Jr. *Modern Clinical Syphilology.* Philadelphia, W. B. Saunders Company, 1944.

ANDREW JACKSON

Andrews, E. Benjamin. "The Oregon Question," *Encyclopedia Americana,* 1943.

Bassett, John Spencer. *The Life of Andrew Jackson.* New York, The Macmillan Company, 1908.

Cecil, Russell L. *A Textbook of Medicine.* 8th ed. Philadelphia, W. B. Saunders Company, 1951.

Editorial, "Primary Amyloidosis," *Journal of the American Medican Association,* Vol. CXL, No. 9 (July 2, 1949).

Gardner, Frances Tomlinson. "The Gentleman from Tennessee," *Surgery, Gynecology, and Obstetrics,* Vol. LXXXVIII, No. 3 (March, 1949).

Jaffe, R. H. *Pathological Conference.* Evanston, Ill., Cook County Internes' Association, 1940.

James, Marquis. *Andrew Jackson: A Portrait of a President.* New York, Literary Guild, 1933.

Mayo Clinic. *Collected Papers of Mayo Clinic and Mayo Foundation,* Vol. XXIV. Philadelphia, W. B. Saunders Company, 1933.

Parton, James. *Life of Andrew Jackson.* 3 vols. Boston, Fields, Osgood and Company, 1870.

Year Book of General Medicine. Chicago, Year Book Publishers, 1939.

JOHN PAUL JONES

Cecil, Russell L. *A Textbook of Medicine.* 8th ed. Philadelphia, W. B. Saunders Company, 1951.

Ficarra, Bernard J. "Eleven Famous Autopsies in History," *Annals of Medical History*, 3 Ser., Vol. IV (November, 1942), 504–20.

Johnson, Gerald W. *The First Captain.* New York, Coward-Mc-Cann, Inc., 1947.

Russell, Paul F., Luther F. West, and Reginald D. Manwell. *Practical Malariology.* 1st ed. Philadelphia, W. B. Saunders Company, 1946.

Russell, Phillips. *John Paul Jones.* New York, Brentano's, 1927.

Tooker, L. F. *John Paul Jones.* New York, The Macmillan Company, 1916.

IMMANUEL KANT

Friedman, E. D. "Affections of the Blood Vessels of the Brain." In *A Textbook of Medicine*, 6th ed., by Russell L. Cecil. Philadelphia, W. B. Saunders Company, 1946.

Greene, Theodore Meyer. *Kant—Selections.* New York, Charles Scribner's Sons, 1929.

Stuckenberg, John H. W. *The Life of Immanuel Kant.* London, The Macmillan Company, 1882.

Wasianski, E. A. Car, and Thomas De Quincy. "Immanuel Kant," in *Great Short Biographies of Ancient Times*, compiled by Barrett H. Clark. New York, Albert and Charles Boni, 1932.

JOHN KEATS

Brandenburgh, Albert Jaques. *Life of John Keats.* Trans. from the French by J. Middleton Murray. New York, Peter Smith, 1929.

British Authors of the Nineteenth Century. New York, H. W. Wilson Company, 1936.

Colvin, Sir Sidney. *Keats.* In English Men of Letters series. London and New York, The Macmillan Company, 1887.

Lowell, Amy. *John Keats.* 2 vols. Boston and New York, Houghton Mifflin Company, 1925.

Osler, William. *An Alabama Student and Other Essays.* New York, Oxford University Press, 1906.

Severn, Joseph. Articles in *The Atlantic Monthly*, April, 1863.

NANCY HANKS LINCOLN

Beveridge, Albert J. *Abraham Lincoln.* 4 vols. New York, Houghton Mifflin Company, 1928.

Bulger, Harold A., Francis M. Smith, and Orlius Steinmeyer. "Milk Sickness and the Metabolic Disturbances in White Snakeroot Poisoning," *Journal of the American Medical Association*, Vol. XCI, No. 25 (December 22, 1928).

Cecil, Russell L. *A Textbook of Medicine.* 6th ed. Philadelphia, W. B. Saunders Company, 1946.

Couch, James Fitton. "Milk Sickness, the Result of Richweed Poisoning," *Journal of the American Medical Association*, Vol. XCI, No. 4 (July 28, 1928).

Muenscher, Walter Conrad. *Weeds.* New York, The Macmillan Company, 1936.

Nicolay, John G., and John Hay. *Abraham Lincoln.* 2 vols. New York, The Century Company, 1894.

Pommel, L. H. *A Manual of Poisonous Plants.* Cedar Rapids, Iowa, Torch Press, 1909.

Smith, Harvey H. *Lincoln and the Lincolns.* Springfield, Ill., Pioneer Publications, 1931.

Stern, Philip Van Doren. *The Life and Writings of Abraham Lincoln.* New York, Random House, 1940.

Thienes, Clinton H. *Clinical Toxicology.* Philadelphia, Lea and Febiger, 1940.

Wright, A. M. R. *The Dramatic Life of Abraham Lincoln.* New York, Grossett and Dunlap, 1925.

JEAN PAUL MARAT

Andrews, George Clinton. *Diseases of the Skin.* Philadelphia, W. B. Saunders Company, 1946.

Burr, C. W. "Jean Paul Marat, Physician, Revolutionist, Paranoiac," *Annals of Medical History*, Vol. II (Fall, 1919), 248–61.

Ormsby, Oliver S., and Hamilton Montgomery. *Diseases of the Skin*. Philadelphia, Lea and Febiger, 1948.

Queries and Minor Notes, *Journal of the American Medical Association*, Vol. CI, No. 10 (September 2, 1933).

Tobias, Norman. *Essentials of Dermatology*. Philadelphia, J. B. Lippincott Company, 1941.

Wells, H. G. *The Outline of History*. New York, Garden City Publishing Company, 1929.

GUY DE MAUPASSANT

Cecil, Russell L. *A Textbook of Medicine*. 8th ed. Philadelphia, W. B. Saunders Company, 1951.

Hardin, E. B. "Paresis of Guy de Maupassant," *Journal of the American Medical Association*, Vol. LXIX (November 3, 1917), 1555.

Maupassant, Guy de. *"Le Horla,"* in *Great Tales of Horror and the Supernatural*, compiled by Herbert A. Wise and Phyllis Fraser. New York, Random House, 1944.

Roz, Firmin. "Guy de Maupassant," in *Warner Library*, XVI, 9803–9808. 30 vols. New York, Knickerbocker Press, 1917.

Steegmuller, Francis. *Maupassant: A Lion in the Path*. New York, Random House, 1949.

Stokes, John H., Herman Beerman, and Norman Ingraham. *Modern Clinical Syphilology*. Philadelphia, W. B. Saunders Company, 1944.

WILLIAM McKINLEY

Buffalo Evening Express, September 6, 1901 ff.

Buffalo News and Telegraph, September 6, 1901 ff.

Editorial, *American Medicine*, Vol. II, No. 11 (September 14, 1901), 391.

———. Vol. II, No. 12 (September 21, 1901), 779.

Editorial, *Journal of the American Medical Association*, Vol. XXXVII, No. 16 (October 19, 1901), 1040.

Ficarra, Bernard J. "Eleven Famous Autopsies of History," *An-*

nals of Medical History, 3 Ser., Vol. IV (November, 1942), 518–19.

Rixey, P. M., Matthew D. Mann, and Others. "Official Report on the Case of President McKinley," *Journal of the American Medical Association*, Vol. XXXVII, No. 16 (October 19, 1901), 1029–36.

NAPOLEON BONAPARTE

Bainville, Jacques. *Napoleon*. Trans. from the French by Hannah Miles. New York, Little, Brown and Company, 1933.

Bechet, P. E. "Napoleon: His Last Illness and Post-mortem," *Bulletin* of the New York Academy of Medicine, Vol. IV (April, 1928), 469.

Cecil, Russell L. *A Textbook of Medicine*. 8th ed. Philadelphia, W. B. Saunders Company, 1951.

Ludwig, Emil. *Napoleon*. New York, Boni and Liveright, Inc., 1926.

Sokolov, Boris. *Napoleon: A Doctor's Biography*. New York, Prentice-Hall, Inc., 1927.

Vincent, Esther H. "The Cancer of Destiny," *Surgery, Gynecology, and Obstetrics*, Vol. LXXXVI (January, 1948), 119.

SIR ISAAC NEWTON

Bell, E. T. *Men of Mathematics*. New York, Simon and Schuster, 1937.

Brewster, Sir David. *Memoirs of the Life, Writings, and Discoveries of Sir Isaac Newton*, Edinburgh, T. Constantine and Company, 1855.

Figuier, Louis. "Sir Isaac Newton," Lives of Illustrious Scientists, in *Great Short Biographies of Modern Times*, compiled by Barrett H. Clark. New York, Albert and Charles Boni, 1932.

More, Louis T. *Isaac Newton*. New York, Charles Scribner's Sons, 1934.

SAMUEL PEPYS

Duke-Elders. *Textbook of Ophthalmology*. St. Louis, C. V. Mosby, 1949. Vol. IV, p. 42–61.

Ficarra, Bernard J. "Eleven Famous Autopsies in History," *An-*

nals of Medical History. 3 Ser., Vol. IV (November, 1942), 507.

MacLauren, C. *Post-Mortems of Mere Mortals*. New York, Doubleday, Doran and Company, 1935.

Pepys, Samuel. *Diary*. 2 vols. With notes by Richard, Lord Braybrook. London, I. M. Dent and Sons, Ltd., 1906.

———. *Diary*. With additions by H. B. Wheatley. New York, E. P. Dutton and Company, 1908.

Power, D'Arcy. "Medical History of Mr. and Mrs. Samuel Pepys," *Lancet* (London), June 1, 1895.

PETER THE GREAT

Graham, Stephen. *Peter the Great*. New York, Simon and Schuster, 1929.

Grinker, Roy. *Neurology*. Springfield, Ill., Charles C. Thomas, 1945.

Motley, John Lothrop. "Peter the Great," in *Great Short Biographies of Modern Times*, compiled by Barrett H. Clark. New York, Albert and Charles Boni, 1932.

Oudard, George. *Peter the Great*. Trans. from the French by F. M. Atkinson. New York and London, Payson and Clark, Ltd., 1930.

Penfield, Wilder, and Theodore Erickson. *Epilepsy and Cerebral Localization*. Springfield, Ill., Charles C. Thomas, 1945.

Purvis, Stewart, Sir James. *The Diagnosis of Nervous Diseases*. Baltimore, Williams and Wilkins, 1945.

Tempkin, Owser. *Falling Sickness*. Baltimore, The John Hopkins Press, 1945.

Veastinoya, Nais. *Peter the Czar*. Hollywood, David Graham Fisher, 1919.

Waliszewski, K. *Peter the Great*. Tr. from the French by Lady Mary Loyd. New York, D. Appleton and Company, 1897.

Wight, O. W. *Life of Peter the Great*. 2 vols. Boston, Houghton Mifflin Company, 1882.

PHILIP II

Cecil, Russell L. *A Textbook of Medicine*. Philadelphia, W. B. Saunders Company, 1951.

Hench, Philip S. "Diagnosis and Treatment of Gout and Gouty Arthritis," *Journal of the American Medical Association*, Vol. CXVI (1941), 453.

Hume, Martin A. S. *Life of Philip II of Spain*. New York, The Macmillan Company, 1897.

Loth, David. *Philip II of Spain*. New York, Brentano's, 1932.

Myers, Philip Van Ness. *Mediaeval and Modern History*. New York, Ginn and Company, 1905.

———. "Spain," in *New Larned History*, IX, 7920–22. 12 vols. Springfield, Mass., C. A. Nichols Publishing Company, 1923.

Prescott, William Hickling. *History of the Reign of Philip the Second, King of Spain*. 2 vols. Boston, Phillips, Sampson and Company, 1858–59.

Turner, Edward Raymond. *Europe 1450–1789*. New York, Doubleday, Page and Company, 1925.

 EDGAR ALLAN POE

Allan, Carlisle. "Cadet Edgar Allan Poe, U. S. A.," *American Mercury*, August, 1933.

Allen, Hervey. *Israfel: The Life and Times of Edgar Allan Poe*. 2 vols. New York, Rinehart, 1927.

Karnosh, Louis J. "The Insanities of Famous Men," *Journal of the Indiana State Medical Association*, Vol. XXIX, No. 1 (January, 1936), 8.

Reaser, Edward F. "Edgar Allan Poe: A Psychiatric Case Study," *West Virginia Medical Journal*, Vol. XXXVI, No. 2 (February, 1940), 73–80.

ROBERT LOUIS STEVENSON

Balfour, Graham. *The Life of Robert Louis Stevenson*. 2 vols. New York, Charles Scribner's Sons, 1908.

Bermann, Richard A. *Home From the Sea*. Trans. from the German by Elizabeth Reynolds Hapgood. Indianapolis and New York, Bobbs-Merrill Company, 1939.

Editorial, "Robert Louis Stevenson," *Detroit Medical Journal*, Vol. XVIII (June, 1917), 234–38.

Editorial, *Journal of the American Medical Association*, Vol. CXLII (March 4, 1950), 654.

Kunitz, Stanley, and Howard Craycraft. *British Authors of the Nineteenth Century*. New York, H. W. Wilson Company, 1936.

Moorman, Lewis J. *Tuberculosis and Genius*. Chicago, University of Chicago Press, 1940.

DEAN SWIFT

Abstracts of Current Medical Literature, *Journal of the American Medical Association*, Vol. CXXXVIII (December 11, 1938), 1120.

Ballenger, W. L. *Diseases of the Nose, Throat, and Ear*. 9th ed. Philadelphia, Lea and Febiger, 1947.

Dandy, Walter E. "Ménière's Disease," *Proceedings* of the Interstate Post-graduate Medical Association of North America, Vol. XI (October, 1935), 248–51.

Katz, Benjamin. "Ménière's Syndrome," *Annals of Western Medicine and Surgery*, Vol. III, No. 10 (October, 1949).

Sholl, Ann McClure. "Jonathan Swift," in *Warner Library*, XXXIII, 14259–64. 30 vols. New York, Knickerbocker Press, 1917.

Van Doren, Carl. *The Portable Swift*. New York, Viking Press, 1948.

Wilson, T. G. "Dean Swift," *Annals of Medical History*, 3 Ser., Vol. II (May 10, 1940).

GEORGE WASHINGTON

Fay, Bernard. *George Washington*. Boston and New York, Houghton Mifflin Company, 1931.

Ford, Paul Leicester. *The True George Washington*. Philadelphia, Lippincott, 1896.

Hay, James, Jr. "Washington's Conquest of Physical Handicaps," *Hygeia*, Vol. IX (August, 1931), 736.

Mitchell, S. W. *Youth of Washington*. New York, The Century Company, 1904.

Sparks, Jared. *Life of George Washington*. Boston, Tappan, 1844.

Wells, W. A. "Last Illness and Death of Washington," *Virginia Medical Monthly*, January, 1927.

WALT WHITMAN

Burroughs, John. *Walt Whitman: A Study*. New York, Houghton Mifflin Company, 1906.

———. "Walt Whitman," in *Warner Library*, XXVI, 15885–91. 30 vols. New York, Knickerbocker Press, 1917.

Dictionary of American Biography. New York, Charles Scribner's Sons, 1943.

Kunitz, Stanley J., and Howard Craycraft. *American Authors, 1600–1900*. New York, H. W. Wilson Company, 1938.

Rogers, Cameron. *The Magnificent Idler*. New York, Doubleday, Page and Company, 1926.

Trent, Josiah C. "Walt Whitman: A Case Study," *Surgery, Gynecology, and Obstetrics*, Vol. LXXXVII, No. 1 (July, 1948).

Whitman, Walt. "When Lilacs Last in the Dooryard Bloomed," in *Great Poems of the English Language*, compiled by Wallace Alvin Briggs. New York, Tudor Publishing Company, 1933.

Winwar, Frances. *American Giant*. New York, Harper and Brothers, 1941.

WILLIAM THE CONQUEROR

Bigham, Hon. Clyde. *The Kings of England*. New York, E. P. Dutton and Company, 1929.

Freeman, Edward A. *William the Conqueror*. New York, The Macmillan Company, 1907.

Gardiner, Samuel R. *Student's History of England*. New York, Longmans, Green and Company, 1929.

Gardner, Frances Tomlinson. "Bells Toll for Primes: An Inquiry into the Fate of William the Conqueror," *Surgery, Gynecology, and Obstetrics*, Vol. LXXXVI, No. 3 (March, 1948).

Green, John Richard. *A Short History of the English People*. New York, American Book Company, 1916.

Stenton, Frank Merry. *William the Conqueror*. New York, G. P. Putnam's Sons, 1925.

SUPPLEMENTARY BIBLIOGRAPHY

Howard F. Stein

Bloch, Marc L. B. *The Royal Touch: Sacred Monarchy and Scrofula in England and France* (translation of Les Rois Thaumaturges). London, Routledge and Kegan Paul, 1973.

Brady, F. *James Boswell: The Later Years, 1769–1795.* New York, McGraw-Hill, 1984.

Feder, Stuart. "Gustav Mahler, Dying," *International Review of Psycho-Analysis* 5 (1978):125–48.

Freud, Sigmund. "Dostoevsky and Parricide," *The Standard Edition of the Complete Psychological Works of Sigmund Freud (SE)* 21 (1928): 175–96. London, Hogarth Press, 1961.

Freud, Sigmund. "Psycho-Analytic Notes on an Autobiographical Account of a Case of Paranoia," *SE* 12 (1911):3–82. London, Hogarth Press, 1958.

Friedlander, W. J. "About 3 Old Men: An Inquiry into How Cerebral Arteriosclerosis Has Altered World Politics: A Neurologist's View (Woodrow Wilson, Paul von Hindenburg, and Nikolai Lenin)," *Stroke* 3 (July–Aug. 1972):467–73.

Hart, G. D. "The Habsburg Jaw," *Canadian Medical Association Journal* 104 (April 3, 1971):601–603.

Hodge, G. P. "A Medical History of the Spanish Habsburgs, as Traced in Portraits," *Journal of the American Medical Association* 238 (11) (Sept. 12, 1977):1169–74.

Loevy, H. T., and A. Kowitz. "The Habsburgs and the 'Habsburg Jaw,'" *Bulletin of the History of Dentistry* 30 (1)(April 1982):19–23.

Niederland, William. *The Schreber Case: Psychoanalytic Profile of a Paranoid Personality.* New York, Quadrangle/The New York Times Book Co., 1974.

Peele, Stanton. "The Life Study of Alcoholism: Putting Drunkenness in Biographical Context (James Boswell)," *Bulletin of the Society of Psychologists in Addictive Behaviors* 5 (1) (1986): 49–53.

Schatzman, Morton. *Soul Murder: Persecution in the Family.* New York, The New American Library, 1976.

Shaw, Peter. "All in the Family: A Psychobiography of the Adamses," *The American Scholar* 54 (4) (Autumn 1985): 501–16.

Stierlin, Helm. *Adolf Hitler: A Family Perspective.* New York, Psychohistory Press, 1976.

Weisman, Avery D., and Robert K. Kastenbaum. *The Psychological Autopsy.* New York, Human Sciences Press, 1968.

INDEX